2nd Edition

PARAMEDIC
CRASH COURSE®

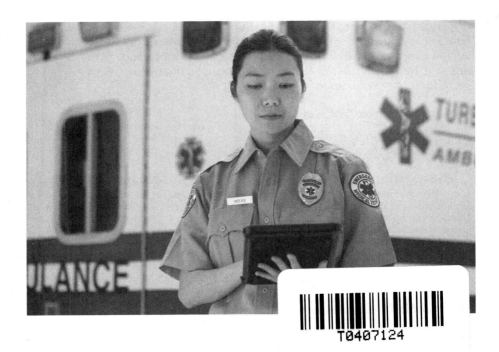

Chris Coughlin, PhD, NRP, NEMSEC

Research & Education Association
www.rea.com

Research & Education Association
1325 Franklin Ave., Suite 250
Garden City, NY 11530
Email: info@rea.com

PARAMEDIC CRASH COURSE®, 2ND EDITION

Copyright © 2025 by LSC Communications Book LLC d/b/a Research & Education Association, a division of Lakeside Book Company. Prior edition copyright © 2019 by Research & Education Association. All rights reserved. No part of this book may be reproduced in any form without permission of the publisher.

Printed in the United States of America

ISBN-13: 978-0-7386-1288-1
ISBN-10: 0-7386-1288-X

LIMIT OF LIABILITY/DISCLAIMER OF WARRANTY: Publication of this work is for the purpose of test preparation and related use and subjects as set forth herein, and is published based on available information as of the publication date, understanding that such information and practices may change over time. While every effort has been made to achieve a work of high quality, neither Research & Education Association nor the authors and other contributors of this work guarantee the accuracy, currentness, or completeness of or assume any liability in connection with the information and opinions contained herein and in REA's software and/or online materials. REA and the authors and other contributors shall in no event be liable for any personal injury, property or other damages of any nature whatsoever, whether special, indirect, consequential or compensatory, directly or indirectly resulting from the publication, use or reliance upon this work. Neither REA nor the author is engaged in nor shall be construed as offering legal, nursing or medical advice or assistance or a plan of care. If legal, nursing, or medical assistance is required, the services of a competent professional person should be sought. Links to external sites in this publication or companion online materials are provided as a convenience to readers and for informational purposes only. Though every reasonable effort has been made to publish current links, URLs may change over time. No endorsement of any external link is made or implied, and neither the publisher nor the author(s) are responsible for the accuracy, legality, or content of any external site or for that of subsequent links. All trademarks cited in this publication are the property of their respective owners.

NREMT and National Registry of Emergency Medical Technicians are trademarks of the National Registry of Emergency Medical Technicians, which neither sponsors nor endorses this product. All other trademarks cited in this publication are the property of their respective owners.

Cover image: © gettyimages.com/JeffreyMarkowitz

 REA Crash Course® and REA® are registered trademarks of Research & Education Association.

C25

Table of Contents

Chapter 8: Pulmonology 133
Chapter 9: Neurology 145
Chapter 10: Endocrinology 157
Chapter 11: Anaphylaxis 167

PART V

MEDICAL EMERGENCIES (PART 2)
Plus review questions

Chapter 12: Gastrointestinal/Genitourinary 175
Chapter 13: Toxicology 185
Chapter 14: Hematology and Infectious Disease 203
Chapter 15: Behavioral Disorders 219
Chapter 16: Eye, Ear, Nose, and Throat Disorders 231
Chapter 17: Musculoskeletal Disorders 237

PART VI

TRAUMA
Plus review questions

Chapter 18: Soft Tissue and Orthopedic Injuries 243
Chapter 19: Burn Injuries 253
Chapter 20: Head and Spinal Injuries 265
Chapter 21: Chest, Abdomen, and Pelvic Injuries 279
Chapter 22: Environmental Emergencies 291

PART VII

SPECIAL PATIENTS
Plus review questions

Chapter 23: Obstetrical and Gynecological Emergencies 309
Chapter 24: Neonatology 327
Chapter 25: Pediatrics 339
Chapter 26: Geriatrics 355
Chapter 27: Special Patient Populations 365

Paramedic Crash Course
TABLE OF CONTENTS

About Our Author v
About REA v
About Our Book vi
Preface vii
Acknowledgments viii

Anatomy & Physiology Review .... *www.rea.com/paramedic*

PART I — INTRODUCTION
Getting Started xi

PART II — PHARMACOLOGY
Plus review questions

Chapter 1: Medication Administration/Drug Calculations 3
Chapter 2: Drug Profiles 15

PART III — AIRWAY/ASSESSMENT/BLEEDING AND SHOCK
Plus review questions

Chapter 3: Airway/Oxygenation/Ventilation 51
Chapter 4: Patient Assessment 67
Chapter 5: Patient Monitoring Technology 85
Chapter 6: Bleeding and Shock 99

PART IV — MEDICAL EMERGENCIES (PART 1)
Plus review questions

Chapter 7: Cardiology and Resuscitation 115

ABOUT OUR BOOK

REA's fully revised and updated second edition of *Paramedic Crash Course* is designed for the last-minute studier or any prospective candidate seeking a quick refresher before taking the National Paramedic Certification Exam. This *Crash Course* review shows you how to study efficiently and strategically, providing the edge you need to pass the exam.

Written by a veteran EMS Program Director and NREMT paramedic, the book contains the following targeted content, including 150 end-of-chapter review questions:

- **Part I** offers an overview of the exam, outlining the topics covered, as well as tips for reducing stress in the run-up to the exam and on test day.

- **Part II** reviews pharmacology and includes advice for avoiding medication administration errors and a look at drug calculations.

- **Part III** covers airway, patient assessment, and bleeding and shock.

- **Parts IV and V** cover medical emergencies.

- **Part VI** reviews trauma, including environmental emergencies.

- **Part VII** is devoted to special patients through the prism of obstetrical and gynecological emergencies; neonatology; pediatrics; and geriatrics.

- **Part VIII** reviews EMS operations, including ground and air ambulance operations; incident management; and rescue operations, hazmat, and terrorism.

Additional online resources, available at *www.rea.com/paramedic*, include the following:

- **Anatomy & Physiology Review.** This section meets you where are with a handy reference for A&P. To help you integrate your test prep, A&P subjects are flagged throughout the book.

- **Paramedic References.** The book comes with a comprehensive list of outside resources to enrich your command of the subject matter.

ABOUT OUR PRACTICE EXAM

Are you ready for the exam? Find out by taking REA's digital practice exam available at *www.rea.com/studycenter*. This practice test features automatic scoring and explains every answer. Let it pinpoint your strengths and weaknesses so you'll be ready on exam day.

Good luck on your Paramedic national certification exam!

PART VIII — EMS OPERATIONS
Plus review questions

Chapter 28: Ground and Air Ambulance Operations 377
Chapter 29: Incident Management 385
Chapter 30: Rescue Operations, Hazardous Materials, Terrorism 393

ANSWERS TO REVIEW QUESTIONS 411

ONLINE PRACTICE EXAM .... *available at www.rea.com/studycenter*

REFERENCES .... *www.rea.com/paramedic*

ABOUT OUR AUTHOR

Dr. Chris Coughlin is Paramedic Studies Program Director at Contra Costa College in San Pablo, California. Dr. Coughlin is a nationally certified EMS instructor. In 2006, he became one of the first 850 nationally certified flight paramedics (FP-C) in the United States. He previously worked as a critical care flight paramedic in Phoenix, and served as the Department Chair of Public Safety Sciences at Glendale Community College in Glendale, Arizona. He is also the author of REA's acclaimed *EMT Crash Course*.

Dr. Coughlin has degrees in Paramedicine from Glendale Community College, Adult Education from Ottawa University, and Educational Leadership from Northern Arizona University. He holds a doctorate in Educational Philosophy from Capella University.

Dr. Coughlin welcomes correspondence at *ccoughlin@contracosta.edu*.

ABOUT REA

Founded in 1959, Research & Education Association (REA) is dedicated to publishing the finest and most effective educational materials—including study guides and test preps—for students of all ages.

Today, REA's wide-ranging catalog is a leading resource for students, teachers, and other professionals. Visit *www.rea.com* to see our complete catalog.

A LETTER FROM OUR AUTHOR

This book is intended for current paramedic students and recent graduates who will be sitting for the national certification exam. Your primary paramedic text is probably 2,000+ pages and impossible to memorize. This completely revised and updated *Paramedic Crash Course* is not meant to replace that resource. Nonetheless this *Crash Course* review is considerably more concise than your paramedic text (good news) and focuses on providing you with the must-know information needed to pass the certification exam. This book doesn't contain everything; however, you need to know just about everything in it. The book is based on a few presumptions:

1. You are completing, or have completed, a high-quality programmatically accredited paramedic education program.

2. You completed a human anatomy & physiology course either before or during your paramedic education program.

3. You are proficient at ECG interpretation.

4. You are knowledgeable about the current American Heart Association guidelines for Basic Life Support and Advanced Cardiac Life Support.

Listen carefully to any advice provided by your paramedic education program core instructors, program director, and medical director. These experts know you, your strengths and weaknesses, and your dominant learning style. Your program also has access to information regarding how its graduates have historically performed on the certification exam. Their NREMT pass rates are most likely available on the National Registry website, or upon request.

You should be able to review this book, memorize the material you agree is important and don't already know, and complete the included practice exam in 30 days or less. The good news is you don't need to be an academic all-star or a brilliant test-taker to do well on the national certification exam (most of us who passed this exam are neither of those things). You just need a genuine desire to help others and a strong work ethic.

Study hard. Good luck. Be safe!

Chris Coughlin
PhD, NRP, NEMSEC

AUTHOR DEDICATION AND ACKNOWLEDGMENTS

Dedicated to my children, Saren, Alissa, Hannah, and Nathan, who I am proud to watch as they pursue their own paths; and to my wife, Lisa, who I would travel any path with.

Special thanks to the following technical reviewers:

Aaron Bates
EMT Program Director
Contra Costa College

Rainier Perez
EMS Program Director
Glendale Community College

PUBLISHER'S ACKNOWLEDGMENTS

Publisher: Pamela Weston

Editorial Director: Larry B. Kling

Technical Editors: Aaron Bates and Rainier Perez

Copy Editor: Sally Fay

Digital Content Prep: Heidi Gagnon

Book File Prep: Jennifer Calhoun

Typesetting: Caragraphics

PART I
INTRODUCTION

Getting Started

Passing the national paramedic certification exam lets the public, employers, and state licensing authorities know that you have demonstrated competency. The NREMT exam is a pass/fail test that is rigorous, comprehensive, and highly effective at assessing entry-level competency.

This section is designed to do three things:

1. Demystify the exam. If you know what to expect, you can be better prepared.
2. Provide specific information and tips to help you prepare and reduce your stress level.
3. Identify essential content you need to know to pass the exam.

THE EXAM

The NREMT exam is a computer-adaptive test (CAT) that utilizes sophisticated software to assess and adapt to your individual abilities. This means that everyone will feel challenged by the test. The exam delivers one question at a time, and the questions are *not* randomly chosen. With each answer you submit, the test recalibrates its estimate of your ability level. The estimate gets more precise as the exam progresses. The exam ends when there is 95% certainty that your competency level is either above or below the passing standard.

You will have 3.5 hours to complete the exam which, because it is adaptive, will present between 110 and 150 questions. Don't worry about running out of time. More than 99% of candidates finish the exam in the time allowed. The exam is based on the National EMS Scope of Practice Model, the National EMS Education Standards, the National Registry Practice Analysis, and the current American Heart Association Guidelines for Cardiopulmonary Resuscitation and Emergency Cardiovascular Care.

This means correct answers on the exam are based on national standards, not local protocols or any one textbook. The NREMT intentionally avoids regionally specific or controversial content.

You will likely find most of the questions on the NREMT exam to be relevant and fair. Every question is referenced to a task in the NREMT Practice Analysis. Each correct answer is confirmed to be accurate and current. The correct answers reflect what's contained in commonly available EMS textbooks. Each test question that affects your score will have spent about one year in the development process. In addition to scored questions, paramedic candidates will see about 20 "pilot" questions on the test that are still in the development process. Pilot questions are indistinguishable from scored items; however, they will not count toward your score.

Typically, you can access your test results through the NREMT website within two business days after completing the exam. Rest assured: *This book arms you with all the advice and information you need to pass the test*; however, those who don't are provided limited information about their performance to help them prepare to retake the test. Candidates must wait at least 14 days before retaking the exam. The NREMT charges an exam fee for each attempt.

The NREMT website provides a great deal of information about the examination and certification process. For additional information about the NREMT exam, visit *www.nremt.org*.

The NREMT complies with the Americans with Disabilities Act (ADA) of 1990 by offering reasonable testing accommodations for individuals with disabilities.

TOPICS COVERED ON THE EXAM

NREMT Exam Topics	Distribution of Questions
Airway, Respiration & Ventilation	9%–13%
Cardiology & Resuscitation	11%–15%
Trauma	7%–11%
Medical/Obstetrics/Gynecology	25%–29%
EMS Operations	6%–10%
Clinical Judgment	31%–35%

Source: National Registry of Emergency Medical Technicians

Getting Started

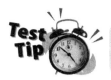

Test Tip: You will see questions about pediatric patients throughout the exam. Think of pediatric assessment/emergencies as the "seventh category" on the test.

QUESTION FORMATS

The NREMT has expanded the types of questions on the paramedic certification exam. There will be plenty of traditional multiple-choice questions; however, the exam will also include technology-enhanced items that use computer technology designed to better simulate clinical practice.

MULTIPLE-RESPONSE ITEM QUESTIONS

You may see some multiple-choice questions with five answer choices that have two correct answers. Other multiple-choice questions may have six answer choices that ask you to select three correct answers. The exam will always tell you when a question requires more than one answer choice.

SCENARIO-BASED ITEMS

The paramedic exam includes scenario-based items designed to deeply assess the candidate's knowledge and skills related to clinical judgment. Such items focus on the en-route, on-scene, and post-scene components of an EMS call. NREMT believes that these items will more accurately reflect what you will experience in the field and will allow you to demonstrate the decision-making process experienced during comprehensive patient care activities. Each of these scenario-based items will include up to 10 questions. Paramedic candidates will see at least two of these scenario-based sets with up to 10 questions each.

Don't stress over question formats you may not have seen before. You will get some practice with them throughout the chapters in this book and on the included online practice test. You can also see sample questions and YouTube videos created by the National Registry by visiting https://www.nremt.org/Document/TEIs.

xiii

Introduction

PREPARING FOR THE TEST

- NREMT exams are delivered by Pearson VUE. Instructions for scheduling your exam are available at *www.nremt.org*. Candidates can test at any authorized Pearson VUE testing center in the United States, or from your home or office via the OnVUE online testing system. For more details on your testing options, visit *https://www.pearsonvue.com/us/en/nremt/onvue.html*.

- Thoroughly prepare for the test. There is no other way to pass.

- Expect questions that test your clinical judgment, critical thinking, and knowledge of pathophysiology, not just fact recall. About 35% of the exam will be focused on clinical judgment.

- Read this book. This book is an important tool in your preparation, but it should not be the only tool.

- Review the current American Heart Association Guidelines for Cardiopulmonary Resuscitation and Emergency Cardiovascular Care. You *will* be tested on this information at the paramedic level.

- Use reliable practice questions to identify your areas of strength and weakness. Dedicate additional time to identified areas of potential weakness.

- Do *not* memorize specific questions you think will be on the test. Instead, study the tasks, knowledge, skills, and abilities required for entry-level competency. This will equip you to tackle whatever questions await you.

- Apply what you are learning in an active learning format that works for you. This might include flashcards, mental imagery, verbally reciting content, writing exercises, highlighting, practice questions, and study groups.

- Visit *https://www.nremt.org/Document/TEIs* to learn about the various types of questions on the exam.

- Don't procrastinate. Take the test as soon as possible after completing your paramedic program. The longer you wait, the more your chances of passing go down.

- Don't cram. You should be done preparing the day before the test, not beginning to prepare.

- Have an organized study plan and dedicate time to studying every day.

Medication Administration/ Drug Calculations

I. TERMS TO KNOW

A. **Bioavailability:** The amount of a drug that enters central circulation and is able to cause an effect.

B. **Bolus:** Administration of medication in a single dose (as opposed to an infusion).

C. **Concentration:** For calculation purposes, this is the total amount of medication available as packaged, e.g., total amount of drug (mcg, mg, g) in the syringe, ampule, etc.

D. **Dose:** The drug amount intended for administration.

E. **Enteral:** Delivery of medication through the gastrointestinal (GI) tract (oral, sublingual, rectal).

F. **Parenteral:** Delivery of medication outside of the GI tract, e.g., intravenous (IV), intraosseous (IO), intramuscular (IM), subcutaneous (SC), intranasal (IN).

G. **Volume:** For calculation purposes, this is the total amount of fluid available as packaged, e.g., total amount of fluid (mL) in the syringe, ampule, etc.

II. MEDICATION LEGISLATION

A. **Pure Food and Drug Act (1906):** Prevents manufacture, sale, or transportation of misbranded or poisonous medications.

B. **Harrison Narcotic Act (1914):** Regulated production, importation, and distribution of opiates.

Chapter 1

    C. Federal Food, Drug, and Cosmetic Act (1938): Gives U.S. Food and Drug Administration authority to oversee the safety of food, drugs, and cosmetics.

    D. Controlled Substances Act (1970): Categorized controlled substances based on their potential for abuse and potential medical benefits.

        1. Schedule I substances
   - i. High potential for abuse. No accepted medical use.
   - ii. Examples: heroin, LSD, ecstasy, peyote.

        2. Schedule II substances
   - i. Narcotics and stimulants with high potential for abuse.
   - ii. Examples: methadone, morphine, codeine, methamphetamine, amphetamine, dextroamphetamine.

        3. Schedule III substances
   - i. Less potential for abuse; can still cause low physical or high psychological dependence.
   - ii. Examples: Vicodin, acetaminophen with codeine, ketamine, anabolic steroids.

        4. Schedule IV substances
   - i. Low potential for abuse.
   - ii. Examples: Xanax, Soma, Valium, Ativan, Versed.

        5. Schedule V substances
   - i. Contain limited quantities of narcotics, such as cough syrups with codeine.

III. AVOIDING MEDICATION ERRORS

    A. The Six Rights of Drug Administration
1. Right patient
2. Right drug
3. Right time
4. Right route

PART II
PHARMACOLOGY

- Get plenty of rest the night before the test. Caffeine and energy drinks are not a substitute for a good night's sleep.
- Arrive for the test mentally focused, not tired, hungry, or otherwise distracted. Bring a sweater if you get cold easily.
- If you are already doing shift work, do not work the night before taking the test.
- Know exactly where the testing center is for your scheduled test. Arrive early (not on time) and absolutely do not be late. Bring the required identification.
- You do not need to have extensive computer or typing skills to take the test.
- The test centers are ADA compliant. Visit *www.nremt.org* for additional information about the National Registry's ADA policies.

DURING THE EXAM

- Take a moment to calm your mind and focus on your breathing. Believe in yourself and the work you have put in to make it this far.
- The test will have a clock letting you know how much time you have left. Don't let this distract you. You will finish the test in the time allowed.
- You will have access to an on-screen calculator throughout the test.
- Read each question ... and multiple times if necessary. Each question contains clues to help you identify the correct answer(s). The risk of misreading a question is much greater than the risk of running out of time.
- Irrelevant information is eliminated from questions before you see them. The information in the questions is included for a reason.
- When you are torn between two answer choices (and you will be), go with the option that is most beneficial for your patient. When in doubt, treat.
- You cannot skip a question or come back to it later.
- Stay calm. Trust your instincts. Don't get frustrated. You made it this far for a reason. The test will feel hard; however, that does NOT mean that you are failing.

Introduction

AFTER THE EXAM

- Exam results are posted to your NREMT account within two business days. Consider not taking the test on a Friday if you'll stress all weekend waiting for your results.
- To access your results, log in to your NREMT account and click on the "Dashboard" or "My Application."

5. Right amount
6. Right documentation

B. Keep similarly packaged drugs separated in drug box, such as ampules of epinephrine and morphine.

C. Always confirm medication and dose with fellow emergency medical services (EMS) provider.

D. If you pull it or draw it up, you administer it.

E. Confirm dosage with appropriate reference sources (American Heart Association guidelines, state standards, agency protocols, etc.).

F. Most medications should be stored within a temperature range of 59°F to 86°F.

G. Medications should be kept in a secure location and stored according to manufacturer's recommendations.

IV. COMMON PREHOSPITAL ROUTES OF MEDICATION ADMINISTRATION

A. Enteral (through the GI tract)
 1. Oral
 2. Rectal

B. Parenteral (outside of the GI tract)
 1. Subcutaneous
 2. Intramuscular
 3. Intravenous
 4. Intraosseous
 5. Sublingual
 6. Buccal
 7. Nasal
 8. Inhaled

Chapter 1

V. MEDICATION PACKAGING

A. Ampules

B. Vials (single-dose and multidose)

C. Prefilled syringes

D. Reconstitution-required meds, e.g., glucagon

E. IV fluids
   1. Colloids
   2. Crystalloids
      i. Ringer's lactate
      ii. 0.9% sodium chloride (aka normal saline)
      iii. Dextrose 5%

VI. DRUG CALCULATIONS

A. Metrics review
   1. Liter (measure of volume)
      i. 1,000 milliliters (mL) = 1 liter (L)
      ii. *Note:* 1 mL = 1 cubic centimeter (cc).
   2. Gram (measure of weight)
      i. 1,000 micrograms (mcg or μg) = 1 milligram (mg)
      ii. 1,000 mg = 1 gram (g)
      iii. 1,000 g = 1 kilogram (kg)
      iv. 1 kg = 2.2 pounds (lb)

B. Bolus calculations
   1. (Volume of fluid in mL × desired sodium chloride dose in mg) ÷ Concentration (the total amount of drug as packaged) = mL to administer
      i. Above formula can also be expressed as: $\dfrac{V \times D}{C} = mL$

ii. **Example 1:** You are ordered to administer 0.5 mg of atropine using a 1 mg/10 mL syringe.

Volume = 10 mL

Dose = 0.5 mg

Concentration = 1 mg

$$\frac{10 \times 0.5}{1} = 5 \text{ mL}$$

iii. **Example 2:** You are ordered to administer 1 mg per kg of lidocaine to a 50 kg patient using a 100 mg/5 mL syringe.

Volume = 5 mL

Dose = 50 mg (50 kg × 1)

Concentration = 100 mg

$$\frac{5 \times 50}{100} = 2.5 \text{ mL}$$

iii. **Example 3:** You are ordered to administer 2 mg of diazepam using a 10 mg/2 mL syringe.

Volume = 2 mL

Dose = 2 mg

Concentration = 10 mg

$$\frac{2 \times 2}{10} = 0.4 \text{ mL}$$

C. IV infusions
   1. IV tubing drop factors (drops per mL)
      i. Macrodrip tubing = typically 10 drops per mL (may also be 15 or 20)
      ii. Microdrip (pediatric) tubing = 60 drops per mL
   2. IV infusion calculations (no medications added)
      i. $$\frac{\text{Ordered volume (mL)} \times \text{IV tubing drop factor}}{\text{Minutes}} = \text{drops per minute}$$
      ii. **Example 1:** 150 mL per hour with macrodrip tubing

      Ordered vol = 150

      Drop factor = 10

Chapter 1

   Minutes = 60

   $$\frac{150 \times 10}{60} = 25 \text{ drops per min}$$

   iii. **Example 2:** 65 mL per hour with microdrip tubing

   Ordered vol = 65

   Drop factor = 60

   Minutes = 60

   $$\frac{65 \times 60}{60} = 65 \text{ drops per min}$$

D. IV medication infusions (medication added to IV bag)

1. $$\frac{\text{Volume of IV bag} \times \text{Dose of med ordered} \times \text{Tubing drop factor}}{\text{Concentration (total amt of drug in IV bag)} \times \text{Minutes}} = \text{drops per min}$$

2. **Example 1:** Administer 2 mg per minute of lidocaine with microdrip tubing using 1 g (1,000 mg) of lidocaine in 250 mL IV.

   Volume = 250 mL

   Dose = 2

   Tubing = 60

   Concentration = 1,000 (dose is in mg, so concentration must also be in mg)

   Minutes = 1

   $$\frac{250 \times 2 \times 60}{1,000 \times 1} = 30 \text{ drops per min}$$

3. **Example 2:** Administer 5 mcg per kg per minute of dopamine using microdrip tubing with 400 mg of dopamine in 250 mL IV. Patient weight is 90 kg.

   Volume = 250

   Dose = 450 (90 kg × 5)

   Tubing = 60

   Concentration = 400,000 (Dose and concentration must both be in mg or mcg. Can't have one in mg and the other in mcg.)

   Minutes = 1

   $$\frac{250 \times 450 \times 60}{400,000 \times 1} = 17 \text{ drops per min}$$

VII. DRUG CALCULATIONS REVIEW FLASHCARDS

Calculations	
How many mcg (μg) per mg?	1,000 mcg (μg) per mg
How many mg per gram?	1,000 mg per g
How many pounds per kg?	2.2 lbs per kg
How many mL per liter?	1,000 mL per L
What is the drop factor for: ➤ Blood tubing ➤ Macro (Adult) tubing ➤ Pediatric tubing	**Blood** (a "macro" tubing) = 10 drops per mL **Macro (not blood)** aka "regular" or "adult" tubing = Variable drip rate (10, 15, 20 drops per mL) **Pediatric** "micro" tubing = 60 drops per mL
What is the abbreviation for drop and drops?	Drop = gtt Drops = gtts
What is the formula for calculating a bolus medication?	$$\frac{\text{Volume} \times \text{Dose}}{\text{Concentration}} = \text{mL needed}$$ Ex: Give 3 mg of valium — Volume = 2 mL Packaging: 10 mg in 2 mL — Dose = 3 mg Concentration = 10 mg (2 × 3) ÷ 10 = **0.6 mL**
What is the formula for calculating a plain IV infusion rate?	$$\frac{\text{Ordered Volume} \times \text{Drop Factor}}{\text{Minutes}} = \text{Drops per minute}$$ Ex: 100 mL per hour with 10 drop tubing (100 × 10) ÷ 60 = **17 drops per min**

|9

Chapter 1

What is the formula for calculating an IV medication infusion?	$$\frac{\text{Volume} \times \text{Dose} \times \text{Drop Factor}}{\text{Concentration} \times \text{Minutes}} = \text{Drops per minute}$$		
	Ex: Give 5 mcg/kg/min of dopamine (90 kg patient) **Pkg:** 400 mg in 250 mL	Volume = 250 mL Dose = 450 mcg (5 × 90) Tubing = 60 (peds) Concentration = 400 mg Minutes = 1		
	Note: The dose and concentration must match (both mg or both mcg). You can convert dose from 450 mg to .450 mcg or convert concentration from 400 mg to 400,000 mcg.		
	(250 × .450 × 60) ÷ (400 × 1) = **17 drops per min**		

Practice: Plain IV Infusions

Use 60 gtts peds tubing for 1–5:	Use 10 gtts blood tubing for 6–10:	Use 15 gtts adult tubing for 11–15:
1) 110 mL/hr	6) 110 mL/hr	11) 110 mL/hr
2) 65 mL/hr	7) 65 mL/hr	12) 65 mL/hr
3) 80 mL/hr	8) 80 mL/hr	13) 80 mL/hr
4) 200 mL/hr	9) 200 mL/hr	14) 200 mL/hr
5) 150 mL/hr	10) 150 mL/hr	15) 150 mL/hr

1) 110 gtts/min	6) 18 gtts/min	11) 28 gtts/min
2) 65 gtts/min	7) 11 gtts/min	12) 16 gtts/min
3) 80 gtts/min	8) 13 gtts/min	13) 20 gtts/min
4) 200 gtts/min	9) 33 gtts/min	14) 50 gtts/min
5) 150 gtts/min	10) 25 gtts/min	15) 38 gtts/min

What are the shortcuts for plain IV flow rate calculations?	As long as the order is over an hour, divide it by: ➤ 6 for blood tubing ➤ 4 for adult (15 gtts) tubing ➤ 1 for peds tubing
	100 mL per hr (blood tubing) = 100 ÷ 6 = **17 drops/min**
	100 mL per hr (adult tubing) = 100 ÷ 4 = **25 drops/min**
	100 mL per hr (peds tubing) = 100 ÷ 1 = **100 drops/min**

Medication Administration/Drug Calculations

Practice: Bolus Calculations

1) atropine 0.5 mg use prefilled syringe	6) atropine 1.2 mg use multidose vial	11) Lasix 80 mg
2) Cordarone 300 mg	7) morphine 2 mg	12) lidocaine 60 mg
3) verapamil 2.5 mg	8) Benadryl 25 mg	13) Valium 2 mg
4) etomidate 24 mg	9) 10 grams of D_{50}	14) calcium 300 mg
5) sodium bicarbonate 20 mEq	10) Succinylcholine 120 mg	15) 1.4 mg epinephrine use 1:1,000 concentration

1) 5 mL	6) 3 mL	11) 8 mL
2) 6 mL	7) 0.2 mL	12) 3 mL
3) 1 mL	8) 0.5 mL	13) 0.4 mL
4) 12 mL	9) 20 mL	14) 3 mL
5) 20 mL	10) 6 mL	15) 1.4 mL

Practice: IV Medication Infusions

Lidocaine Infusions: Use 1g/ 250 mL mix	Epinephrine Infusions: Use 1 mg/ 250 mL mix	Dopamine Infusions: Use 400 mg/ 250 mL mix
1) Lido at 2 mg/min	4) Epi at 4 mcg/min	7) Dopamine 5 mcg/kg/min (90 kg)
2) Lido at 3 mg/min	5) Epi at 6 mcg/min	8) Dopamine 7 mcg/kg/min (90 kg)
3) Lido at 4 mg/min	6) Epi at 8 mcg/min	9) Dopamine 10 mcg/kg/min (90 kg)

Note: Use pediatric (60 gtts) tubing for all problems.

1) 30 gtts/min	4) 60 gtts/min	7) 17 gtts/min
2) 45 gtts/min	5) 90 gtts/min	8) 24 gtts/min
3) 60 gtts/min	6) 120 gtts/min	9) 34 gtts/min

Chapter 1

REVIEW QUESTIONS
(Answers on pg. 411.)

1. Which of the following controlled substances have the highest potential for abuse, with no accepted medical uses?

    A. Schedule I

    B. Schedule II

    C. Schedule III

    D. Schedule IV

2. Which of the following are among the six "rights" of medication administration? (Select THREE.)

    A. the right time

    B. the right protocol

    C. the right route

    D. the right amount

    E. the right certification level

    F. the right cross-check

3. You are ordered to administer 0.5 mg of a medication that is packaged 1 mg in 10 mL. You should administer:

    A. 1 mL.

    B. 0.5 mL.

    C. 5 mL.

    D. 10 mL.

4. Your patient weighs 165 lb. This equals:

    A. 363 kg.

    B. 75 kg.

    C. 80 kg.

    D. 100 kg.

Medication Administration/Drug Calculations

5. What is the drop factor for microdrip (pediatric) tubing?
    A. 10 drops per mL
    B. 15 drops per mL
    C. 20 drops per mL
    D. 60 drops per mL

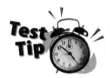

Good news! You will have access to an on-screen digital calculator during the national certification exam.

Drug Profiles

Chapter 2

I. TERMS TO KNOW

A. **Adrenergic:** Related to the sympathetic nervous system (think adrenaline).

B. **Adverse effect:** Unintended effect of a medication administration.

C. **Agonist:** Medication that stimulates a specific response.

D. **Analgesic:** Medication that reduces pain.

E. **Antagonist:** Medication that inhibits a specific action.

F. **Bolus:** Single dose of medication, given all at once.

G. **Cholinergic:** Related to the parasympathetic nervous system (think acetylcholine).

H. **Contraindication:** Circumstance when a medication should not be used.

I. **Drug class:** Categorization of medications that work in the same way or are used to treat the same condition.

J. **Extrapyramidal side effects:** Tremors, slurred speech, restlessness, muscle twitching, anxiety; any effect(s) caused by a medication other than the intended effect(s).

K. **Hypersensitivity:** Undesirable reactions produced by the normal immune system, including allergies and autoimmunity.

L. **Indication:** Circumstance when a medication should be considered.

Chapter 2

   M. **Mechanism of action (MOA):** Pharmacological effects of a medication.

   N. **Refractory:** Resistant to treatment.

   O. **Side effect:** Any unwanted effect of medication administration.

SOURCES OF INFORMATION

   A. United States Pharmacopeia (USP)

   B. National Formulary (NF)

   C. Physician's Desk Reference (PDR)

   D. Drug package inserts

   E. State EMS authority

DRUG CATEGORIES AND INCLUDED DRUGS

   A. Altered level of consciousness (ALOC)/overdose (OD)
      1. Activated charcoal
      2. Dextrose
      3. Glucagon
      4. Nalmefene
      5. Naloxone
      6. Thiamine

   B. Analgesics
      1. Acetaminophen
      2. Fentanyl
      3. Ketorolac
      4. Morphine
      5. Nitrous oxide

C. Antidysrhythmics
   1. Adenosine
   2. Amiodarone
   3. Atropine
   4. Diltiazem
   5. Lidocaine
   6. Verapamil

D. Cardiac
   1. Aspirin
   2. Bumetanide
   3. Dopamine
   4. Epinephrine
   5. Furosemide
   6. Nitroglycerin

E. Electrolytes
   1. Calcium
   2. Magnesium sulfate
   3. Sodium bicarbonate

F. Hemorrhage/misc.
   1. DuoDote
   2. Ondansetron
   3. Oxygen
   4. Oxytocin
   5. Phenylephrine
   6. Promethazine
   7. Tranexamic acid

G. Respiratory
   1. Albuterol
   2. Atrovent

3. Dexamethasone
4. Diphenhydramine
5. Methylprednisolone

H. Sedation/seizure/paralytic
1. Diazepam
2. Etomidate
3. Ketamine
4. Lorazepam
5. Midazolam
6. Olanzapine
7. Succinylcholine

IV. DRUG PROFILE INFORMATION

A. Drug name

B. Drug class/mechanism of action

C. Indications

D. Contraindications

E. Adverse effects

F. Dose
1. *Note:* Drug dosages can vary widely by region.
2. The sample pharmacology thumbnails included in this chapter include recommended dosages; however, they will not likely be an exact match for all regions. Always defer to local protocols regarding use of medications.
3. Reduced dosages often apply to patients with renal or hepatic disease.

Drug Profiles

V. RECEPTOR SITES

A. Alpha 1: Medications that stimulate alpha 1 receptor sites cause vasoconstriction.

B. Beta 1: Medications that stimulate beta 1 receptor sites cause increased heart rate (chronotrope), increased cardiac force of contraction (inotrope), and increased myocardial conduction (dromotrope).

C. Beta 2: Medications that stimulate beta 2 receptors cause bronchodilation.

D. Opioid: Medications that stimulate opioid receptor sites cause central nervous system (CNS) depression and analgesia.

VI. SAMPLE PHARMACOLOGY THUMBNAILS

A. *Note:* Pharmacology protocols can vary widely based on agency, region, medical direction, state protocols, etc. These flashcards are meant to provide a sample of the drug profile information paramedic candidates are typically expected to know.

B. *Always* follow local guidelines regarding administration of medications.

VII. COMMONLY PRESCRIBED MEDICATIONS OF IMPORTANCE

A. Commonly prescribed antidepressants
   1. Amitriptyline (Elavil)
   2. Amoxapine (Asendin)
   3. Aripiprazole (Abilify)
   4. Bupropion (Wellbutrin)
   5. Citalopram (Celexa)
   6. Duloxetine (Cymbalta)
   7. Escitalopram (Lexapro)

8. Fluoxetine (Prozac)
9. Imipramine (Tofranil)
10. Isocarboxazid (Marplan)
11. Nortriptyline (Pamelor)
12. Paroxetine (Paxil)
13. Quetiapine (Seroquel)
14. Selegiline (Emsam)
15. Sertraline (Zoloft)
16. Tranylcypromine (Parnate)
17. Trazodone (Dysyrel)
18. Venlafaxine (Effexor)

B. Commonly prescribed beta-blockers
1. Atenolol (Tenormin)
2. Metoprolol (Lopressor)
3. Propranolol (Inderal)
4. Labetalol
5. Carvedilol

C. Commonly prescribed anticoagulants
1. Apixaban (Eliquis)
2. Dabigatran (Pradaxa)
3. Edoxaban (Savaysa)
4. Enoxaparin (Lovenox)
5. Heparin
6. Rivaroxaban (Xarelto)
7. Warfarin (Coumadin, Jantoven)

D. Commonly prescribed erectile dysfunction (ED) medications
1. Avanafil (Stendra)
2. Sildenafil (Viagra)
3. Tadalafil (Cialis)
4. Vardenafil (Levitra)

ACTIVATED CHARCOAL

Name(s): Actidose-Aqua

Class: Adsorbent

MOA: Reduces systemic absorption of toxins from GI tract

Packaging: 15, 25, 50 g bottle

Indications: Recently ingested toxins

Contraindications
- Ingestion of caustics or hydrocarbons
- Decreased LOC
- Unstable airway

Adverse Reactions
- Nausea & vomiting
- Black stool

Dose
- Adult: 1–2 g per kg (usual dose 30–60 g)
- Pediatric: 0.5–1 g per kg
- *Note:* Caution using activated charcoal that contains sorbitol.

ADENOSINE

Name(s): Adenocard

Class: Antidysrhythmic, endogenous nucleoside

MOA: Slows conduction through AV node, interrupts re-entry pathways, slows sinus rate

Packaging: 6 mg/2 mL vial or prefilled syringe

Indications
- SVT (not A-flutter or A-fib)
- Monomorphic wide complex tachycardia of unknown origin unresponsive to amiodarone or lidocaine

Contraindications
- Sick sinus syndrome
- 2nd-degree or 3rd-degree AV block
- A-fib and A-flutter
- *Note:* Caution in patients with asthma; those on theophylline, Persantine, or Tegretol; and cardiac transplant patients.

Adverse Reactions
- Cardiovascular (CV): Transient asystole, bradycardia, PVCs, palpitations, chest pain, hypotension
- Respiratory: Dyspnea, hyperventilation, tightness in throat, bronchospasm
- Central Nervous System (CNS): Dizzy, lightheaded, headache, paresthesias, blurred vision
- Gastrointestinal (GI): Nausea, metallic taste

Adult Dose
- Initial: 6 mg rapid IV push with immediate 20 mL flush. AC vein preferred. Use port closest to patient, elevate arm during admin. Continuous ECG monitoring required.
- Repeat: May repeat at 12 mg in 1–2 minutes if needed.

Special Considerations
- Short half-life (5 seconds)
- Administer rapidly followed by immediate 20 mL flush
- Reoccurrence of tachydysrhythmia is common

ALBUTEROL

Name(s): Proventil, Ventolin

Class: Sympathomimetic, bronchodilator

MOA: Bronchodilation, decreases airway resistance

Packaging: 2.5 mg/3 mL unit dose (sulfite-free)

Indications: Bronchospasm

Contraindications
- Hypersensitivity
- *Note:* Use caution in combination with other sympathomimetics due to potentiating effects.

Adverse Reactions
- Cardiovascular (CV): Dysrhythmias, tachycardia
- Central Nervous System (CNS): Tremors, nervous, restless

Adult Dose
- 2.5 mg in 3 mL unit dose via SVN or in-line with BVM
- May repeat per medical direction
- May be combined with ipratropium

AMIODARONE

Name(s): Cordarone

Class: Antidysrhythmic

MOA: Negative chronotrope, dilates coronary arteries

Packaging: 150 mg/3 mL ampules or prefilled syringe (50 mg/mL)

Indications
- VF/pulseless VT unresponsive to defib & epinephrine
- Wide complex tachycardia of unknown origin
- Stable VT, SVT, A-fib, A-flutter
- Polymorphic V-tach

Contraindications
- Hypersensitivity
- Bradycardia
- 2nd-degree or 3rd-degree block
- Cardiogenic shock
- Hypotension
- Pulmonary edema, CHF

Adverse Reactions
- Cardiovascular (CV): Bradycardia, hypotension, asystole, AV block, CHF, polymorphic V-tach, prolonged QT interval
- Gastrointestinal (GI): Nausea & vomiting
- Other: Fever, headache, dizziness, flushing, salivation, photophobia

Adult Dose: Cardiac arrest
- 300 mg IV/IO first dose
- Repeat 150 mg IV/IO in 3–5 minutes if still in VF or pulseless VT

Adult Dose: Tachydysrhythmias (v-tach, wide complex tach, A-flutter, A-fib, SVT)
- 150 mg in 50 mL IV bag of D5W IV bag infused over 10 minutes

Adult Dose: Maintenance infusion
- 1 mg per minute IV infusion
  - Ex: Add 150 mg to 50 mL D5W. Run at 20 gtts/min with pediatric tubing **OR**
  - Ex: Add 50 mg to 50 mL D5W. Run at 60 gtts/min with pediatric tubing.

ASPIRIN

Name(s): Acetylsalicylic acid, Bufferin, ASA
Class: Analgesic, antipyretic, anti-inflammatory
MOA: Decreased platelet aggregation
Packaging: 81 & 325 mg tablets

Indications
- Suspected MI (chest pain, ECG changes)
- Unstable angina
- Pain, discomfort, or fever in adult patient only

Contraindications
- Hypersensitivity
- Bleeding ulcer, hemorrhage, hemophilia
- Allergy to salicylates or other NSAIDs
- Children and adolescents

Adverse Reactions
- Use caution in patients with history of asthma
- Side effects rare in adults with single dose

Adult Dose
- Cardiac: 162–324 mg (2–4 pediatric chewables)
- *Note:* ASA has been linked to Reye's syndrome in pediatric patients.
- *Note:* ASA should not be used for suspected stroke without prior cerebral imaging.

ATROPINE

Name(s): Atropine
Class: Anticholinergic, parasympathetic blocker, parasympatholytic
MOA: Increased HR, decreased mucus production, bronchodilation
Packaging: 1 mg/10 mL prefilled syringe (0.1 mg/mL); 8 mg/20 mL multidose vial (0.4 mg/mL)

Indications
- Symptomatic bradycardia
- Organophosphate poisoning

Contraindications
- Hypersensitivity
- Acute angle-closure glaucoma (relative contraindication)

Adverse Reactions
- Tachydysrhythmias
- Ventricular irritability
- Angina
- Dry mouth

Adult Dose: Symptomatic bradycardia
- 1 mg rapid IV push
- Can repeat as needed to a max dose of 3 mg

Adult Dose: Organophosphate poisoning
- 2–5 mg IV, repeat every 5 min as needed (no max dose)
- 8 mg/20 mL multidose vial:
  - 1 mL = 0.4 mg
  - 2.5 mL = 1 mg

Pediatric Dose: Bradycardia
- You MUST correct hypoxia first!
- Atropine is 3rd line for pediatrics and neonates (O_2 and epi first!)
- 0.02 mg/kg (min. 0.1 mg) IV push
- Max single dose: child: 0.5 mg

Special Considerations
- Administering too-small doses or administering too slowly may cause paradoxical bradycardia.
- Not a cardiac arrest drug.
- Use multidose vial for organophosphate, nerve agent.
- Likely ineffective with 2nd-degree type 2 or 3rd-degree AV block.

DEXTROSE

Name(s): D10 (10% solution)
Class: Carbohydrate, hyperglycemic
MOA: Increases blood glucose levels, short-term osmotic diuresis
Packaging: 1 g per 10 mL (Ex: 25 g/250 mL)

Indications
- Known hypoglycemia
- Altered LOC, coma, or seizures of unknown etiology
- Hyperkalemia (in combination with sodium bicarbonate and calcium chloride)

Contraindications
- Head injury
- *Note:* Do **not** withhold dextrose from stroke or traumatic brain injury (TBI) patients with known hypoglycemia.

Adverse Reactions
- Cerebral edema
- Increased ICP
- Tissue necrosis (if IV infiltrates)

Adult Dose
- 12.5–50 g IV
- *Note:* Many jurisdictions now recommend D10 instead of D50 for all patients due to risk of hyperglycemia, cerebral edema, and tissue necrosis.

Pediatric Dose (1 month – 14 years)
- 0.5–1 g per kg of D10 solution over 20 min. To make/admin D10:
  - Remove 50 mL from 250 mL IV bag and add 50 mL of D50
  - Administer 5–10 mL per kg of D10

DIAZEPAM
Name(s): Valium

Class: Benzodiazepine

MOA: CNS depressant, anticonvulsant, sedation

Packaging: 10 mg/2 mL prefilled syringe (5 mg per mL)

Indications
- Grand mal (generalized) seizures
- Transient sedation for medical procedures
- Delirium tremens
- Status epilepticus

Contraindications
- Hypersensitivity
- Angle-closure glaucoma (relative)

Adverse Reactions
- Cardiovascular (CV): Bradycardia, hypotension
- Respiratory: Respiratory depression
- Central Nervous System (CNS): Confusion, coma
- Other: Burning at injection site, tissue necrosis from infiltration

Adult Dose
- IV: 2 mg increments slow IV push (do not exceed 2 mg per min)
- *Note:* For 10 mg/2 mL **packaging:** quickly calculate mL by doubling dose and moving decimal once left. Ex:
  - 2 mg = 0.4 mL
  - 6 mg = 1.2 mL

Pediatric Dose
- IV: 0.2–0.3 mg/kg over at least 3 min or until seizure subsides.
- Rectal (<6 years): 0.3–0.5 mg/kg rectally (slow)

DILTIAZEM

Name(s): Cardizem

Class: Calcium channel blocker

MOA: Negative inotrope, slows SA and AV conduction

Packaging: 5 mg per mL vials

Indications
- A-fib & A-flutter with rapid ventricular rate
- SVT refractory to adenosine

Contraindications
- Hypersensitivity
- Hypotension
- MI or cardiogenic shock
- V-tach
- 2nd-degree or 3rd-degree AV block
- WPW and sick sinus syndrome
- Beta-blockers

Adverse Reactions
- Cardiovascular (CV): Hypotension, bradycardia, AV block, chest pain, asystole
- Gastrointestinal (GI): Nausea & vomiting
- Central Nervous System (CNS): Headache, fatigue, drowsiness

Adult Dose
- Initial dose: 0.25 mg/kg (usually 20 mg) slow IV push over 2 min.
- If no response: repeat in 15 min 0.35 mg/kg (usually 25 mg)
- Consider reduced dose for elderly patients
- *Note:* Consider pretreatment with calcium chloride to reduce possible hypotension.

DIPHENHYDRAMINE

Name(s): Benadryl

Class: Antihistamine, anticholinergic

MOA: Blocks histamine receptors, reduces capillary permeability, reduces vasodilation and bronchospasm, antiemetic

Packaging: 50 mg/1 mL vial

Indications
- Anaphylaxis (after epi)
- Extrapyramidal symptoms
- Nausea & vomiting (consider ondansetron)

Contraindications
- Hypersensitivity
- Angle-closure glaucoma (relative)
- Asthma (relative)
- Nursing mothers

Adverse Reactions
- Cardiovascular (CV): Hypotension, palpitations, dysrhythmias
- Respiratory: Anaphylaxis, thickening bronchial secretions, wheezing
- Central Nervous System (CNS): Sedation, seizures
- Children: Paradoxical CNS excitation

Adult Dose: 25–50 mg slow IV or deep IM

DOPAMINE

Name(s): Intropin

Class: Sympathomimetic

MOA

— 1–2 mcg/kg/min: Cerebral & renal vasodilation, increased urine output

— 2–10 mcg/kg/min: Stimulation of beta 1 receptors for increased heart rate, cardiac output, and BP

— 10–20 mcg/kg/min: Alpha effects, peripheral vasoconstriction, increased PVR & preload

Packaging: 400 mg/5 mL vial (must be added to 250 mL IV fluid) **OR** 400 mg/250 mL premix bag

Indications

— Symptomatic bradycardia (not first line)

— Hemodynamically significant hypotension without hypovolemia (after fluid therapy)

Contraindications: Hypovolemic shock

Adverse Reactions

— Cardiovascular (CV): Dysrhythmias, hypotension (low dose), hypertension

— Gastrointestinal (GI)/Genitourinary (GU): Nausea & vomiting, renal shutdown at higher doses

— Other: Tissue necrosis from infiltration

Adult Dose

— Mix: 400 mg in 250 mL (1,600 mcg/mL)

— Start at 5–20 mcg/kg/min

Special Considerations

— 10% of patient's weight (in lb) is roughly the drops per minute for 5 mcg/kg/min

- Ex: 120 lb patient at 5 mcg/kg/min is about 12 drops per minute (exact = 10.2 gtts/min)

— Use 60 gtts (pediatric) tubing

EPINEPHRINE

Name(s): Adrenalin

Class: Sympathomimetic, adrenergic

MOA
- alpha: Peripheral vasoconstriction
- $beta_1$: Positive inotrope, chronotrope, dromotrope
- $beta_2$: Bronchodilator
- Clinical effects: Increases cerebral & myocardial perfusion; increases HR, BP, & myocardial electrical activity; reverses bronchospasm, anaphylaxis

Packaging
- 1:10,000: 1 mg/10 mL prefilled syringe
- 1:1,000: 1 mg/1 mL amp & 30 mg/30 mL multidose vial

Indications
- Cardiac arrest: All causes
- Severe bronchospasm
- Anaphylaxis
- Symptomatic bradycardia (not first line)
- Hypotension (nonhypovolemic causes)

Contraindications
- None for cardiac arrest
- Hypothermia (relative)

Adverse Reactions
- Cardiovascular (CV): Hypertension, dysrhythmia, tachycardia, angina
- Central Nervous System (CNS): Agitation, anxiety
- Gastrointestinal (GI)I: Nausea & vomiting

Adult Dose: Cardiac arrest
- IV: 1 mg 1:10,000 q 3–5 min followed by 20 mL flush. No max dose.
- ETT: 2–2.5 mg of 1:1,000 diluted to 10 mL

Adult Dose: Hypotension, bradycardia
- 2–10 mcg/min infusion titrate to effect
- 10 mcg/mL q 3–5 min as needed (push-dose epi)

Adult Dose: Asthma, anaphylaxis
- 0.3–0.5 mg 1:1,000 IM preferred (can also administer SC or inject SL)

Pediatric Dose
- IV/IO initial dose for cardiac arrest or refractory bradycardia: 0.01 mg/kg of 1:10,000 (0.1 mL/kg)
- ET initial dose for cardiac arrest or refractory bradycardia: 0.1 mg/kg of 1:1,000 diluted with NS to 3–5 mL (0.1 mL/kg)

Special Considerations
- For epi infusion, 1 mg epi in 250 mL = 4 mcg per mL
- Administer 15 drops per min for every mcg per min. Ex:
  - 1 mcg/min = 15 gtts/min
  - 2 mcg/min = 30 drops/min

FENTANYL
Name(s): Duragesic, Sublimaze
Class: Narcotic analgesic (synthetic)
MOA: CNS depression, pain reliever, decreased preload and afterload

Packaging
- 100 mcg/2 mL **OR** 250 mcg/5 mL
- *Note:* Both are 50 mcg/mL.

Indications
- Analgesia (burns, trauma, MI, renal colic)
- Sedation
- RSI or med-assisted intubation

Contraindications
- Hypersensitivity
- Respiratory depression
- Increased ICP
- Hypotension
- Head injury with altered LOC (relative)
- Asthma (relative)
- Abdominal pain (relative)

Adverse Reactions
- Musculoskeletal: Muscle rigidity (often chest)
- Cardiovascular (CV): Dysrhythmias, hypotension
- Respiratory depression

- Central Nervous System (CNS): Excess sedation, seizures, coma
- Gastrointestinal (GI): Nausea & vomiting

Adult Dose
- IV/IO: 25–50 mcg slow IV push (1–5 min)
- IM: Same as IV/IO (slower onset)
- *Note:* Total dose NOT to exceed 200 mcg.
- *Note:* Respiratory depression may last longer than analgesic.

Pediatric Dose: 1–2 mcg/kg (max 50 mcg)

Special Considerations
- CAUTION: 50–100 times more powerful than morphine.
- Do NOT administer more than 50 mcg (1 mL) in a single dose.

GLUCAGON

Name(s): Glucagon
Class: Pancreatic hormone, hyperglycemic agent
MOA: Converts glycogen to glucose, insulin antagonist
Packaging: 1 mg/1 mL vials (reconstitution required)
Indications: Symptomatic hypoglycemia when IV access is delayed
Contraindications: Hypersensitivity
Adverse Reactions: Nausea & vomiting (rare)
Dose
- Adult (over 44 lb/20 kg): 1 mg IM
- Pediatric: 0.5 mg IM

IPRATROPIUM BROMIDE

Name(s): Atrovent
Class: Anticholinergic, bronchodilator
MOA: Inhibits parasympathetic NS, preferential dilation of larger central airways
Packaging: 500 mcg/2.5 mL unit dose
Indications
- Bronchospasm
- Can be used alone or combined with albuterol

Contraindications
- Hypersensitivity
- Allergy to atropine
- Caution in patients with angle-closure glaucoma

Adverse Reactions
- Respiratory: Cough, increased sputum production
- Central Nervous System (CNS): Dizziness, insomnia, tremors, nervousness
- Gastrointestinal (GI): Nausea

Adult Dose
- 500 mcg in 2.5 mL unit dose via SVN or in-line with BVM
- Can be mixed with albuterol

LIDOCAINE

Name(s): Xylocaine

Class: Antidysrhythmic, local anesthetic

MOA: Increases VF threshold, decreases ventricular irritability

Packaging
- 100 mg/5 mL prefilled syringe (20 mg per mL)
- 1 g/25 mL vial (must be added to 250 mL) **OR** 2 g/500 mL premix bag

Indications
- VT, VF, pulseless VT (amiodarone preferred)
- Maintenance infusion after conversion from VT, VF

Contraindications
- Hypersensitivity
- 2nd-degree or 3rd-degree block
- Do NOT use if heart rate below 60 (treat bradycardia)

Adverse Reactions
- Drowsiness
- Bradycardia
- Paresthesia
- Tinnitus

Chapter 2

Adult Dose: VF, pulseless VT
- Initial bolus of 1–1.5 mg/kg IV push
- Repeat if needed q 5–10 min at 0.5–0.75 mg/kg to max of 3 mg/kg

Adult Dose: Ventricular ectopy with a pulse
- Initial bolus of 0.5–1.5 mg/kg IV push
- Repeat at 0.5–0.75 mg/kg if needed q 5–10 min to max dose of 3 mg/kg

Adult Dose: Maintenance infusion
- Infuse 2–4 mg/min (total mg/kg dose + 1)
- Prepare solution with 1 g in 250 mL NS or 2 g in 500 mL NS for concentration of 4 mg/mL
- Patients over age 70 or with hepatic or renal disease, poor perfusion, CHF: Cut maintenance infusion in half

Special Considerations
- To quickly determine mL for bolus: cut total dose in half and move decimal to left
  - Ex: 60 mg = 3 mL
- Infusion = 15 gtts per min for every mg per min (use 60 gtts tubing)
  - 1 mg/min = 15 gtts/min
  - 2 mg/min = 30 gtts/min
  - 3 mg/min = 45 gtts/min
  - 4 mg/min = 60 gtts/min

LORAZEPAM

Name(s): Ativan

Class: Benzodiazepine

MOA: CNS depression, anticonvulsant

Packaging: 2 mg/mL or 4 mg/mL

Indications
- Seizures, status epilepticus
- Agitated (excited) delirium, also known as hyperactive delirium syndrome with severe agitation

Contraindications
- Hypersensitivity

- Angle-closure glaucoma
- Myasthenia gravis
- Pregnancy (relative)

Adverse Reactions
- Confusion
- Sedation
- Amnesia
- Hypotension
- Respiratory depression

Adult Dose
- Seizures: 2–5 mg slow IV/IO (at least 2 min); max 10 mg
- *Note:* May be given deep IM if no IV/IO access.

Pediatric Dose
- Seizures: 0.05–0.1 mg/kg slow IV/IO (at least 2 min); max 4 mg
- *Note:* May be given deep IM if no IV/IO access.

MAGNESIUM SULFATE

Name(s): Magnesium sulfate, MgSO4

Class: Electrolyte, tocolytic, antidysrhythmic

MOA: Decreases ventricular irritability, inhibits muscular excitability

Packaging: 1 g/2 mL vials

Indications
- Polymorphic V-tach, aka torsades de pointes
- VF/pulseless VT refractory to amiodarone or lidocaine
- Hypomagnesemia
- Preterm labor
- Pregnancy-induced hypertension (pre-eclampsia and eclampsia)
- Severe asthma

Contraindications
- Hypersensitivity
- AV block
- Hypermagnesemia
- Renal impairment

Adverse Reactions
- Cardiovascular (CV): Hypotension, dysrhythmias
- Respiratory: Respiratory depression or paralysis
- Central Nervous System (CNS): Sweaty, drowsy, depressed reflexes
- Gastrointestinal (GI): Nausea
- Other: Flushed
- *Note:* Calcium may help reverse MgSO4 toxicity.

Adult Dose: Cardiac arrest
- VF/pulseless VT: 1–2 g IV over 1–2 min
- Polymorphic VT: 1–2 g IV over 1–2 min followed by 1–2 g over 1 hr
- *Note:* If respiratory rate drops below 12 per min, discontinue MgSO4.

Adult Dose: OB/asthma
- Preterm labor/pre-eclampsia/eclampsia: 4 g in 100 mL over 15 min
- Asthma: 2 g in 50 mL over 5–10 min
- *Note:* If respiratory rate drops below 12 per min, discontinue MgSO4.

MIDAZOLAM
Name(s): Versed
Class: Benzodiazepine
MOA: CNS depression, anticonvulsant, sedation
Packaging: 5 mg/5 mL vial

Indications
- Anticonvulsant
- Sedation
- Facilitation of intubation
- Acute agitation/excited delirium

Contraindications
- Hypersensitivity
- Angle-closure glaucoma
- Neuromuscular disorders (relative)
- Intoxication (relative)
- COPD (relative)

- Respiratory compromise (relative)
- Pregnancy (relative)

Adverse Reactions
- CV: Cardiac arrest, dysrhythmias, hypotension
- Resp: Respiratory depression, wheezing, coughing, hiccups
- CNS: Tremors, drowsiness, headache
- GI: Nausea & vomiting
- *Note:* Respiratory arrest possible when used with narcotics or if administered too rapidly.

Adult Dose
- Sedation: Patients 14–60 years of age
  - 1–10 mg slow IV/IO titrate to effect (max 2.5 mg over 2 min)
  - 2–5 mg IM
- Sedation: Patients over 60 years of age
  - 1–3.5 mg slow IV/IO as above
  - 1–5 mg IM
- Seizures (no IV/IO access): 0.2 mg/kg deep IM

Pediatric Dose
- IV/IO: 0.05–0.1 mg/kg slow push
- IM/IN: 0.2 mg/kg (preferred route for pediatric seizures)

MORPHINE

Name(s): Morphine

Class: Narcotic analgesic

MOA: CNS depression, pain reliever, decreased preload and afterload

Packaging: 10 mg/1 mL ampule or syringe

Indications
- Analgesia (burns, trauma, MI, renal colic)
- Cardiogenic pulmonary edema

Contraindications
- Hypersensitivity
- Respiratory depression
- Hypovolemia
- Hypotension

— Head injury

— Increased ICP

— Asthma (relative)

— Abdominal pain (relative)

Adverse Reactions

— Cardiovascular (CV): Bradycardia, orthostatic hypotension

— Respiratory: Respiratory depression

— Central Nervous System (CNS): Seizures, coma

— Gastrointestinal (GI): Nausea & vomiting

Adult Dose: 1–3 mg slow IVP titrate to effect

NALOXONE

Name(s): Narcan

Class: Narcotic antagonist

MOA: Competitively blocks opioid receptor sites, reverses respiratory depression due to narcotics

Packaging: 0.4 mg ampules, 1 mg/mL prefilled syringe, and 4 mg intranasal spray

Indications

— Narcotic overdose

— Unconscious patient of unknown etiology

Contraindications: Hypersensitivity

Adverse Reactions

— May not reverse histamine effects of narcotic OD

— Withdrawal symptoms

— Combative patient

— Shorter half-life than many narcotics (risk of secondary overdose)

Adult Dose

— IV, ET, IM, SQ, SL: 0.4–2 mg as needed, titrate to effect

— Intranasal: 1 mg each nostril with mucosal atomizer device, repeat as needed

— *Note:* May substitute with nalmefene (Revex) 2 mg.

Pediatric Dose

— Under 5 years of age: 0.1 mg/kg IV, ET, SL, SC, IO

NITROGLYCERIN

Name(s): Nitrostat, NitroMist

Class: Vasodilator, organic nitrate, antianginal

MOA: Decreased preload & afterload, coronary artery vasodilation, increased myocardial oxygen supply, decreased myocardial oxygen demand

Packaging: 0.4 mg tablets or spray

Indications
- Angina
- MI
- CHF with pulmonary edema

Contraindications
- Hypotension
- Hypovolemia
- Increased ICP
- Erectile dysfunction meds (Ex: Viagra, Levitra, Cialis)

Adverse Reactions
- Hypotension
- Reflex tachycardia
- Headache
- Burning under tongue

Adult Dose
- 0.4 mg tablet or spray
- May repeat ×3 with BP over 100 systolic & medical direction approval
- Establish IV access prior to administration

OXYGEN

Name: Oxygen (O_2)

Class: Gas

MOA: Increases tissue oxygenation

Indications
- Cardiac arrest
- Bradycardia in infants/pediatrics

Chapter 2

- Any patient receiving PPV
- Suspected hypoxia, shock, TBI
- SpO$_2$ below 94%

Contraindications: Unsafe conditions

Adverse Reactions
- Hyperoxia
- Possible respiration depression in COPD patients

Dose: Sufficient to maintain SpO$_2$ of at least 94%

OXYTOCIN

Name(s): Pitocin, Syntocin

Class: Hormone, uterine stimulant

MOA: Increases force and frequency of uterine contractions

Packaging: 10 units/1 mL ampule or vial

Indications: Severe postpartum hemorrhage (over 500 mL) within first 24 hrs

Contraindications: Hypersensitivity

Adverse Reactions
- Cardiovascular (CV): Shock, tachycardia
- Respiratory: Anaphylaxis
- Gastrointestinal (GI): Nausea & vomiting

Adult Dose
- 10–20 units in 1,000 mL NS or LR titrate to effect
- Can also administer 10 units IM
- *Note:* Use only after delivery of the placenta.

PROMETHAZINE

Name(s): Phenergan

Class: Antiemetic, antihistamine

MOA: Blocks histamine receptors

Packaging
- 25 mg/1 mL vial
- 50 mg/1 mL vial

Indications
- Nausea & vomiting
- Sedation

Contraindications: Hypersensitivity to Phenergan, Compazine, Thorazine

Adverse Reactions
- Extravasation can cause tissue necrosis
- May lower seizure threshold
- Sedation, drowsiness
- Extrapyramidal symptoms

Adult Dose: Nausea & vomiting
- 12.5 mg IV or deep IM (not SQ!)
- Older patients: 6.25 mg
- Not for children under 2 years old
- Children over 2 years: Consult medical direction
- *Note:* Ondansetron (Zofran) often preferred due to limited side effects and contraindications.

THIAMINE

Name(s): Vitamin B_1, Betalin

Class: Vitamin

MOA: Required for carbohydrate metabolism

Packaging: 100 mg/1 mL ampule or tubex

Indications
- Alcoholism, delirium tremens
- Coma of unknown etiology
- Wernicke-Korsakoff syndrome (thiamine deficiency)

Contraindications: None

Adverse Reactions: Hypotension (rare)

Adult Dose: 100 mg IV or IM

Chapter 2

 VIII. ADDITIONAL PARAMEDIC MEDICATIONS USED IN SOME EMS SYSTEMS

> ➤ *Remember:* According to the NIH, intravenous acetaminophen may offer a similar level of pain relief to opioids, with a lower risk of adverse side effects.

ACETAMINOPHEN
Class: Analgesic
MOA: Antipyretic
Indications: Pain, fever
Contraindications
— Hypersensitivity
— Caution in patients with liver disease
Adverse Effects: Nausea & vomiting (N&V)

CALCIUM
Class: Electrolyte
MOA: Positive inotrope
Indications
— Acute hypocalcemia
— Acute hyperkalemia
— Ca channel blocker OD
— Pretreatment for verapamil or diltiazem
Contraindications
— Hypercalcemia
— Concurrent digoxin therapy (relative)
Adverse Effects
— Asystole
— Bradycardia
— Tissue necrosis on infiltration
— Cardiac dysrhythmias if taking digoxin

DEXAMETHASONE

Name(s): Decadron

Class: Glucocorticoid

MOA: Anti-inflammatory

Indications
- Reactive airway disease
- Asthma
- Anaphylaxis

Contraindications
- Hypersensitivity
- Allergy to sulfa drugs

Adverse Effects
- Edema
- Hypertension
- Convulsions
- Anaphylaxis

DUODOTE/MARK 1

Name(s): Atropine, Pralidoxime

Class: Cholinergic antidote

Indications: Reverse effects of organophosphate/nerve agent exposure

Contraindications: Hypersensitivity

Adverse Effects
- Tachycardia
- Hypertension
- Hyperventilation

KETOROLAC

Name(s): Toradol

Class: NSAID

MOA: Analgesic/antipyretic

Indications: Pain, fever

Contraindications
- Hypersensitivity
- Trauma
- Hemorrhage
- Preop patients
- Labor
- Renal disease
- Patients over 75 years of age

Adverse Effects
- N&V
- GI bleeding
- Heart failure
- Hemorrhagic stroke
- Drowsiness

METHYLPREDNISOLONE
Name(s): Solumedrol
Class: Steroid
MOA:
- Anti-inflammatory
- Stabilizes cell membrane

Indications
- Reactive airway disease
- Anaphylaxis
- Airway burns

Contraindications: Hypersensitivity
Adverse Effects: None from single dose

OLANZAPINE
Name(s): Zyprexa
Class: Antipsychotic
Indications: Acute agitation
Contraindications: Hypersensitivity
Adverse Effects: Respiratory depression

Drug Profiles

ONDANSETRON
Name(s): Zofran
Class: Antiemetic
Indications: N&V
Contraindications
- Hypersensitivity
- Long QT syndrome
- Caution in patients with liver problems

Adverse Effects
- Headache
- Fatigue
- Diarrhea

PHENYLEPHRINE
Name(s): Neo-Synephrine
Class: Topical vasoconstrictor
Indications: Reduce bleeding during nasal intubation
Contraindications: Hypersensitivity
Adverse Effects: None

SODIUM BICARBONATE
Class: Buffer
MOA: Raises pH
Indications
- Metabolic acidosis
- Aspirin or cyclic antidepressant OD
- Cardiac arrest (last line)

Contraindications: Alkalosis
Adverse Effects
- CHF
- Edema
- Intracellular acidosis
- Tissue necrosis on infiltration

SUCCINYLCHOLINE

Name(s): Anectine, Quelicin
Class: Short-acting neuromuscular blocker
MOA: Paralytic
Indications: Facilitation of rapid sequence induction
Contraindications
- Hypersensitivity
- Hyperkalemia
- Malignant hyperthermia
- Penetrating eye injuries
- Airway obstruction
- Neuromuscular disorder
- Epiglottitis
- Burns, crush injury

Adverse Effects
- Prolonged apnea
- Fasciculations
- Hyperkalemia
- Inability to intubate following paralysis

TRANEXAMIC ACID (TXA)

Name(s): Cyklokapron, Lysteda
Class: Hemostatic agent
MOA: Facilitates clotting
Indications: Hemorrhage
Contraindications: Hypersensitivity
Adverse Effects
- Seizures
- Pulmonary embolism
- Headache
- Vision changes

REVIEW QUESTIONS
(Answers on pg. 412.)

1. Which of the following medications has alpha 1, beta 1, and beta 2 effects?
   A. diphenhydramine
   B. epinephrine
   C. diltiazem
   D. lidocaine

2. Ondansetron is indicated for:
   A. nausea and vomiting.
   B. atrial fibrillation.
   C. rapid sequence intubation.
   D. hypoglycemia.

3. Which of the following is a common adverse reaction of IV dextrose administration?
   A. hypoglycemia
   B. decreased intracranial pressure
   C. sedation
   D. tissue necrosis following IV infiltration

4. Diazepam is indicated for:
   A. traumatic brain injury.
   B. hyperkalemia.
   C. generalized seizures.
   D. ventricular tachycardia.

Chapter 2

5. Which of the following is most likely to occur following administration of fentanyl?
   A. CNS depression
   B. CNS excitation
   C. hypertension
   D. muscle paralysis

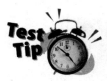

The exam will be full of questions that challenge your patient assessment skills. These are often scenario-based questions. Thoroughly memorize the components of patient assessment, from scene size-up through reassessment. Knowing the order steps and priorities of patient assessment will help guide you to the correct answer!

PART III
AIRWAY/ASSESSMENT/ BLEEDING AND SHOCK

Chapter 3

Airway, Oxygenation, Ventilation

I. TERMS TO KNOW

A. **Angioedema:** Rapid edema of tissue, often in the face, tongue, or larynx.

B. **Cellular respiration:** Cellular processes that convert energy from nutrients into adenosine triphosphate (ATP) and then release waste products.

C. **Exhalation:** The passive part of breathing.

D. **External respiration:** Oxygen exchange between the lungs and circulatory system.

E. **Hypoxia:** Oxygen deficiency.

F. **Inhalation:** The active part of breathing.

G. **Internal respiration:** Oxygen exchange between blood and cells of the body.

H. **Minute ventilation:** Volume of gas inhaled or exhaled per minute (respiratory rate × tidal volume).

I. **Oxygenation:** Delivery of oxygen to the blood.

J. **SVN:** Small volume nebulizer.

K. **Ventilation:** Moving air in and out of the lungs.

Chapter 3

 ANATOMY & PHYSIOLOGY REVIEW

> *Note:* See "Respiratory System" in the online Anatomy & Physiology Review at *www.rea.com/paramedic* for essential information.

 AIRWAY

A. Manual airway techniques come first (as indicated).
   1. Head-tilt, chin-lift (preferred)
   2. Jaw-thrust (suspected spinal injury)

B. Suction comes second (as indicated).
   1. Rigid suction catheters
      i. Used to suction oral airway.
      ii. Aka tonsil tip or Yankauer catheter.
   2. French suction catheters
      i. Used to suction nose, stoma, or inside advanced airway.
      ii. Aka soft-tip, whistle-tip, or flexible catheter.
      iii. Available in numerous sizes (diameters), e.g., 3 French through 40 French. Increased number = increased diameter.
   3. Suction time cannot exceed:
      i. 15 seconds for adults.
      ii. 10 seconds for children.
      iii. 5 seconds for infants.

C. Mechanical airway adjuncts come third (as indicated).
   1. Basic adjuncts
      i. Oropharyngeal airway: For unresponsive patients without a gag reflex (avoid posterior displacement of the tongue).
      ii. Nasopharyngeal airway: Can be used on patients with decreased LOC, but not unresponsive.

2. Advanced airway management
   i. Extraglottic, retroglottic, and supraglottic airway devices
      ➤ Common types used prehospital:
         — Laryngeal mask airway (LMA) and LMA Supreme
         — I-Gel supraglottic LMA
         — Pharyngeal tracheal lumen airway
         — Esophageal tracheal combitube
         — King LT airway
         — Supraglottic airway laryngopharyngeal tube
      ➤ Advantages
         — Easy to use.
         — Blind insertion, no laryngoscope needed.
         — Able to insert quickly (avoid posterior displacement of the tongue).
         — High success rate.
   ii. Endotracheal tube (ETT) intubation
      ➤ Advantages
         — Isolates the trachea.
         — Eliminates gastric distention from ventilation.
         — No mask seal needed.
         — Improved suctioning ability.
         — Route for medication administration (naloxone, epinephrine, atropine, lidocaine).
      ➤ Disadvantages
         — Extensive training required.
         — Direct visualization of vocal cords required.
         — Takes longer than other advanced airways.
         — Has many serious complications.
         — Not been shown to increase survival rates.

- Failure to recognize accidental esophageal intubation will lead to inadequate ventilation and possible brain damage or death.
- *Note:* Following two unsuccessful attempts, switch to another method to secure the airway if possible.

➤ Verification of proper ETT placement
- Direct visualization of cords
- Auscultation of epigastrium and bilateral lung fields
- Continuous waveform capnography
- Pulse oximetry
- Esophageal detector device
- ETT introducer
- *Note:* Inserting the ETT too far into the trachea will likely lead to right mainstem intubation.

iii. Cricothyrotomy (surgical and needle)

➤ Only indicated in acute, life-threatening situations when use of less invasive airway techniques is ineffective.

iv. Rapid sequence induction (intubation) or medication-assisted intubation

➤ Indications
- Respiratory failure
- Inability to protect airway, due to facial trauma, blood, vomit, etc.
- Combative patient, suspected traumatic brain injury
- Persistent hypoxia

➤ Contraindications
- Respiratory and cardiac arrest
- Anticipated difficult airway (relative)
- Short transport time (relative)
- Ability to manage airway with less invasive measures
- Neuromuscular disease, e.g., amyotrophic lateral sclerosis, muscular dystrophy

v. Predictors of difficult advanced airway insertion
- Mouth does not fully open
- Hypersecretions
- Obesity
- Pulmonary edema
- Airway burns
- Facial trauma
- Increased Mallampati score (used with oral intubation)
  — Class I: Entire tonsil clear.
  — Class II: Upper half of tonsil visible.
  — Class III: Soft and hard palate visible.
  — Class IV: Only hard palate visible.

vi. LEMONS mnemonic for difficult airway
- L: Look externally.
- E: Evaluate 3-3-2 rule.
- M: Mallampati score.
- O: Obstruction.
- N: Neck mobility.
- S: Saturations.

IV. OXYGENATION

A. Indications for supplemental oxygen
1. Dyspnea
2. Hypoxia
3. Pulse oximeter below 94%
4. Altered or decreased LOC
5. Respiratory or cardiac arrest
6. Hypoperfusion (shock)

Chapter 3

- B. Supplemental oxygen devices
    1. Nasal cannula
        i. Low-flow oxygen.
        ii. Up to 6 lpm can be administered.
        iii. Delivers 24%–44% oxygen (about 4% per liter above 21% room air).
    2. Nonrebreather (NRB)
        i. High-flow oxygen.
        ii. 10–15 lpm.
        iii. Delivers about 90% oxygen.
    3. Small volume nebulizer (SVN)
        i. Used for delivery of aerosolized medication.
- C. Oxygen cylinders
    1. Cylinder sizes
        i. D cylinder: about 350 L capacity
        ii. E cylinder: about 625 L capacity
        iii. M cylinder: about 3,000 L capacity
    2. Oxygen cylinder pressure
        i. Full cylinder is about 2,000 PSI.
        ii. Safe residual pressure is 200 PSI (cylinder should be taken out of service and refilled once it reaches 200 PSI).
- D. Pin indexing system
    1. Safety feature that prevents an oxygen regulator from being connected to a tank with any other compressed gas, e.g., CO_2 tank
- E. Calculating duration of an oxygen tank
    1. Formula:
    $$\frac{(\text{cylinder PSI} - \text{safe residual pressure}) \times \text{tank constant}}{\text{remaining flow rate (lpm)}} = \text{minutes}$$

2. Tank constants
   i. D cylinder constant: 0.16
   ii. E cylinder constant: 0.28
   iii. M cylinder constant: 1.56
3. Example: You are administering 15 lpm via NRB with a D cylinder oxygen tank with 1,500 PSI remaining.
   (1,300 × 0.16) × 15 = 13.86 minutes

> ***Remember:*** It is critical that you understand when patients need to be oxygenated and when they need to be ventilated. A two-person bag-valve-mask (BVM) ventilation technique is the preferred method of BVM ventilation.

V. VENTILATION

A. Initiate positive pressure ventilation (PPV) for any patient with signs of inadequate breathing, such as:
   1. Excessively bradypneic or tachypneic breathing (age-dependent).
   2. Shallow breathing.
   3. Altered or decreased LOC.
   4. Dyspnea.
   5. Retractions.
   6. Accessory muscle use.
   7. Cyanosis.
   8. Paradoxical motion.
   9. Sucking chest wound.

B. Patients who are breathing fewer than 10 times per minute should be ventilated.

C. When in doubt, ventilate. Patients that don't need it will let you know.

D. *Note:* For out-of-hospital cardiac arrest, BVM ventilation (without intubation) results in the same outcomes as BVM ventilation with advanced airway interventions.

> *Remember:* A National Institutes of Health (NIH) study found that more than 90% of healthcare providers are likely hyperventilating patients with the BVM.

E. Rates of ventilation
  1. Do **not** hyperventilate; it increases the risk of gastric distention, vomiting, aspiration, ineffective CPR, and death.
  2. Adults:
      i. Ventilate at 10 breaths per minute (one breath every 6 seconds).
      ii. *Note:* This includes adult patients with an advanced airway during CPR and those with a pulse who are receiving rescue breathing.
  3. Children and infants:
      i. Ventilate at 20–30 breaths per minute (one breath every 2–3 seconds).
      ii. *Note:* This includes child and infant patients with an advanced airway during CPR and those with a pulse who are receiving rescue breathing.
  4. Newborns:
      i. 40–60 breaths per minute

F. Tidal volumes during PPV
  1. Rise and fall of the chest is an indication of adequate ventilation.
  2. It should take about 1 second to inflate the chest during PPV.

G. Complications of PPV
  1. Increased intrathoracic pressure and reduced cardiac output
  2. Gastric distention and increased risk of vomiting
      i. *Note:* Use of Sellick maneuver (cricoid pressure) to reduce gastric distention is not recommended and should never be used during active vomiting.

Airway, Oxygenation, Ventilation

    H. Automatic transport ventilators (ATVs)

        1. ATVs allow for automated PPV with set rates and tidal volumes.

        2. Tidal volume based on 6–8 mL/kg of ideal body weight.

        3. Advantages:

            i. Very consistent rates and tidal volumes.

            ii. May reduce risk of hyperventilation.

            iii. Allows for hand-free ventilation if advanced airway in place.

        4. Disadvantages

            i. Unable to assess BVM compliance.

            ii. Must base tidal volume on ideal body weight, or risk pulmonary over-pressurization of obese patients.

            iii. Pressure relief valve may prevent effective ventilation in patients requiring higher pressures (disable as indicated).

VI. BREATHING PATTERNS

    A. Agonal respirations

        1. Slow, shallow, infrequent breaths.

        2. Indicates brain anoxia.

    B. Biot's respirations

        1. Irregular pattern of rate and depth and periodic apnea.

        2. Indicates increased intracranial pressure (ICP).

    C. Central neurologic hyperventilation

        1. Deep, rapid respirations.

        2. Indicates increased ICP.

    D. Cheyne-Stokes respirations

        1. Progressively deeper and faster breaths, changing to slower and shallow breaths.

        2. Indicates brain injury.

Chapter 3

E. Kussmaul respiration
1. Deep, gasping breaths.
2. Indicates possible diabetic ketoacidosis.

VII. BREATH SOUNDS

A. Rales (crackles)
1. Fine, bubbling sound on inspiration.
2. Indicates fluid in lower airways.

B. Rhonchi
1. Coarse sounds on inspiration.
2. Indicates inflammation or mucus in lower airways.

C. Wheezes
1. High-pitched sound on inspiration or expiration.
2. Indicates bronchoconstriction.

D. Snoring
1. Indicates partial airway obstruction from the tongue.

E. Stridor
1. High-pitched sound indicating significant upper airway obstruction (e.g., foreign body, angioedema, anaphylaxis).

F. Gurgling
1. Indicates fluid in the upper airway.

VIII. PATIENT MONITORING TECHNOLOGY

A. Pulse oximetry (SpO_2)
1. Measures hemoglobin oxygenation.
2. Can take several minutes to see changes in oxygenation.
3. Can also be used to monitor pulse rate (visual and/or auditory).

4. Should be used with continuous waveform capnography when possible.

B. Capnography (ETCO$_2$)

1. Measures exhaled carbon dioxide and ventilatory status.
2. Reflects changes in ventilatory status almost immediately.
3. Should be used with pulse oximetry when possible.
4. Types of capnography
    i. Capnometry: Provides a numeric display of expired CO$_2$.
    ii. Capnography: Graphic display of capnometry.
    iii. Colorimetric ETCO$_2$: Disposable color-changing device placed between the patient and the ventilation device.
5. Normal arterial CO$_2$ (PaCO$_2$) and ETCO$_2$ values are about 35–45 mmHg.
6. Clinical application of capnography
    i. High ETCO$_2$: Possible hypoventilation.
    ii. Low ETCO$_2$: Possible hyperventilation.
    iii. ETCO$_2$ drops to 0: Possible esophageal intubation or displaced tube.
    iv. Sharp drop in ETCO$_2$: Possible pulmonary embolism, cardiac arrest, hypotension, hyperventilation.
    v. Rapid increase in ETCO$_2$ may indicate return of spontaneous circulation (ROSC).

C. Pulse CO oximetry

1. Newer technology available in prehospital that can detect carboxyhemoglobin and methemoglobin.

IX. CONTINUOUS POSITIVE AIRWAY PRESSURE (CPAP)

A. Indications

1. Indicated for alert and spontaneously breathing patients, at least 12 years of age, in significant respiratory distress, such as sleep apnea, COPD, pulmonary edema, congestive heart failure, pneumonia.

Chapter 3

   2. Candidates for CPAP should demonstrate significant distress, such as tachypnea, SpO_2 below 94%, and/or use of accessory muscles.
   3. Typical starting range: 5–7 cm H_2O.

B. Contraindications
   1. Apnea
   2. Patients unable to follow verbal commands
   3. Suspected pneumothorax
   4. Chest trauma
   5. Tracheostomy
   6. Vomiting
   7. Gastrointestinal bleeding
   8. Hypotension

X. SPECIAL SITUATIONS

> *Remember:* Beware of bradycardia in pediatric patients. Bradycardia in pediatrics is a sign of hypoxia until proven otherwise. Provide supplemental oxygen or PPV as needed to get heart rate up and maintain an SpO_2 of at least 94%.

A. Pediatric patients
   1. Pediatric airway is more easily obstructed.
   2. Infants may need padding under the shoulders. Toddlers may require padding under the head (occiput).
   3. Do not overextend the head and neck. A "sniffing" position is recommended.
   4. Reduce tidal volume to avoid hyperventilation, gastric distention, pulmonary over-pressurization.
   5. Hypoxia develops quickly.
   6. Hypoxia is the most common cause of bradycardia in pediatric patients.

Airway, Oxygenation, Ventilation

    7. Always assume hypoxia in a bradycardic pediatric patient.

    8. Cuffed endotracheal tubes are recommended for all pediatric patients who are being intubated, as it decreases the need for ETT changes.

B. Tracheostomy (trach) tube/stoma

    1. BVM will connect directly to trach tube if one is present.

    2. To ventilate a patient with stoma (no trach tube) use an infant or child mask with appropriate-size BVM. Seal mouth and nose during ventilation.

    3. Trach tubes and stomas require frequent suctioning.

C. Dentures

    1. Dentures are usually secured in place and can be left alone.

    2. If dentures are loose and interfere with airway management or ventilations, they should be removed.

D. Foreign body airway obstruction

    1. Basic life support (BLS)

        i. Conscious adults and children (not infants): Abdominal thrusts or chest thrusts for those who are pregnant or obese.

        ii. Unconscious (all ages): Chest compressions, open airway, look for obstructions, attempt to ventilate, and repeat as needed.

        iii. Conscious infants: Back slaps and chest thrusts.

    2. Advanced life support (when BLS interventions are ineffective)

        i. Attempt to remove foreign body with laryngoscope and McGill forceps.

        ii. Attempt ETT insertion to try passing tube through obstruction or forcing it into right mainstem.

E. Stridor (suspected croup or epiglottitis)

    1. Keep patient calm.

    2. Supplemental oxygen if pulse oximetry below 94%.

    3. Consider saline SVN or nebulized epinephrine (per local protocol).

4. Avoid aggressive airway interventions unless airway becomes completely obstructed.

F. Respiratory burns
   1. Aggressive, early airway intervention is indicated for burn patients with respiratory involvement, e.g., facial burns, stridor, etc.
   2. Consider early intubation due to risk of massive swelling (per local protocol).
   3. *Note:* Any airway swelling evident on initial patient contact **will get worse.**

G. If an airway adjunct must be removed (for example, the patient regains consciousness), have suction immediately available.

H. For patients with gastric distention who are being ventilated, insert an appropriately sized orogastric or nasogastric tube.

REVIEW QUESTIONS
(Answers on pg. 413.)

1. Which of the following is an early indication of hypoxia?
   A. restlessness
   B. decreased LOC
   C. bradycardia
   D. cyanosis

2. Your patient has a pH of 7.30. This indicates:
   A. alkalosis.
   B. hypoxia.
   C. acidosis.
   D. a normal value.

Airway, Oxygenation, Ventilation

3. Inserting the endotracheal tube too far into the trachea will likely result in:

   A. esophageal intubation.

   B. left mainstem intubation.

   C. right mainstem intubation.

   D. tension pneumothorax.

4. Which of the following is a contraindication for rapid sequence induction (RSI)?

   A. respiratory failure

   B. combative patient

   C. persistent hypoxia

   D. respiratory arrest

5. Which of the following are predictive of a difficult intubation? (Select TWO.)

   A. clear view of epiglottis

   B. extremity burns

   C. obesity

   D. hypersecretions

   E. entire tonsil visible

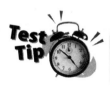

When you get patient care scenarios on the certification exam, **don't hesitate to ventilate!** If you are unsure if you should ventilate your patient, and ventilation is an option, then you probably should.

| 65

Chapter 4

Patient Assessment

I. TERMS TO KNOW

A. **Differential diagnosis:** The process of differentiating between two or more conditions that share similar signs or symptoms.

B. **Field impression:** Field conclusion of the patient's problem based on clinical presentation and exclusion of other possible causes.

C. **Hemostatic dressing:** A dressing or bandage the helps control bleeding by accelerating the clotting process with the help of a clotting agent.

D. **Jaundice:** Yellow discoloration of skin or eyes.

E. **Junctional tourniquet:** Specialized tourniquet used to control bleeding in areas such as inguinal groin or axilla areas.

F. **Marbling/marbled skin:** Pale skin with red/purple patterns.

G. **Mottling/mottled skin:** Patchy appearance to the skin.

H. **Pale/pallor:** Lack of color to skin. Pale may be normal for some people; pallor is an abnormality.

I. **Positive pressure ventilation (PPV):** Artificial ventilation, e.g., bag-valve-mask (BVM).

J. **Primary assessment:** Component of assessment focused on finding and managing immediately life-threatening conditions.

II. OVERVIEW OF PATIENT ASSESSMENT

A. The five major components of patient assessment
   1. Scene size-up
   2. Primary assessment
   3. Patient history
   4. Secondary assessment
   5. Reassessment

B. Patient assessment tips
   1. Patient assessment in the field is not always linear, and you may not get to every component on every patient; however, it helps to think of it in a linear format, as follows:
      i. The scene size-up always comes first and continues throughout the call.
      ii. The primary assessment comes next and precedes all other components of patient assessment.
      iii. The order and priority of the patient history and secondary assessment can change based on the patient's complaint and condition.
      iv. Reassessment is the final step in the assessment process.
   2. Significant trauma patients tend to demand a more intensive primary and secondary assessment and the secondary assessment would take priority over the patient history.
   3. Conscious medical patients often demand a more thorough patient history than some trauma patients and the patient history would take a higher priority than the secondary assessment.
   4. Regardless of the patient's complaint, the patient assessment must be organized and methodical.

C. Methods of forming a field impression
   1. Differential diagnosis based on history and physical exam. Major categories of differential diagnosis include:
      i. Shock.
      ii. Cardiac.

Patient Assessment

      iii. Respiratory.

      iv. Endocrine/metabolic.

      v. Neurologic.

      vi. Infection.

      vii. Gastrointestinal (GI)/genitourinary (GU).

2. Consider past calls and experiences.
3. Gut instinct (sick/not sick).

III. SCENE SIZE-UP

> **Remember:** Know the major components of the scene size-up:
> - Scene safety.
> - Standard precautions.
> - Mechanism of injury (MOI) or nature of illness (NOI).
> - Number of patients.
> - Additional resources.
> - Consider spinal precautions.

A. Scene safety

1. The scene size-up begins as soon as the call is received and doesn't end until the call is over.
2. Rescuers are required to wear an approved high-visibility safety vest at all accident scenes or anytime working near traffic.
3. A portable, impact-resistant, high-intensity flashlight should be carried at all times.
4. Keep your portable radio and cellphone with you whenever possible.
5. Position your emergency vehicle for easy access and to protect the scene if necessary. Never position the loading compartment of the ambulance in the path of oncoming traffic.
6. Some EMS systems will dispatch rescuers to a staging location for a potentially dangerous scene that has not been secured by law enforcement yet. Follow local protocols regarding staging.

- **B.** Standard precautions
  1. Utilize appropriate personal protective equipment (PPE) based on the nature of the call.
  2. Remember to change gloves between patients and before entering the driver compartment of the ambulance to avoid cross contamination.
- **C.** Mechanism of injury (MOI) or nature of illness (NOI)
  1. Understanding the MOI can help predict injury patterns, influence treatment decisions, and help determine hospital destination.
  2. The NOI will be related to the patient's chief complaint, but it is not the same thing, e.g., the patient could have a chief complaint of chest pain, but it could be due to a respiratory problem.
  3. The patient is usually the best source of information; however, at times it will be necessary to question family or bystanders.
  4. Remember, patients can experience both a medical condition and a traumatic injury (Ex: fall due to syncope or vehicle accident due to a seizure).
- **D.** Number of patients
  1. Determine the number of patients.
  2. During a mass casualty incident, do not delay requesting additional resources to get an accurate patient count.
- **E.** Additional resources
  1. Additional resources might include additional advanced life support (ALS) personnel, additional ambulances, special teams, law enforcement, social service resources, etc.
  2. Consider requesting a second apparatus to protect accident scenes in high-traffic areas.
- **F.** Consider spinal precautions
  1. "Spinal immobilization" and associated interventions are no longer part of the national curriculum. Spinal precautions, when needed, are referred to as "spinal motion restriction." See the Head and Spinal Injuries chapter for additional information.
  2. Follow local protocols regarding management of suspected spinal injuries.

IV. PRIMARY ASSESSMENT

> ➤ *Remember:* Know the major components of the primary assessment:
> - General impression.
> - Level of consciousness.
> - ABCs (Airway, Breathing, Circulation).
> - Rapid scan.
> - Transport decision.

A. Primary assessment tips

1. The primary assessment begins as soon as you locate the patient. Remember, the scene size-up is ongoing. You are continuously monitoring and ensuring scene safety, maintaining appropriate PPE, etc.

2. The purpose of the primary assessment is to find and manage immediately life-threatening conditions.

3. The primary assessment may take only seconds in a conscious, stable patient, or you may not be able to move past the primary assessment in a patient with ongoing life threats.

B. General impression

1. The general impression is based on the information you can gather immediately upon encountering the patient or scene.

C. Level of consciousness (LOC)

1. During the primary assessment, the first assessment of LOC is general, not specific.
    i. Conscious and alert?
    ii. Conscious and altered?
    iii. Unconscious?

2. The AVPU scale is used to rapidly determine general responsiveness.
    i. **A** = Alert, e.g., patient's eyes are open and tracking you.
    ii. **V** = Responsive to voice, e.g., "Hey, are you ok?!"

Chapter 4

      iii. **P** = Responsive to pain.

      iv. **U** = Unconscious/unresponsive.

  3. Person, place, time, event (alertness and orientation ×4)

      i. If your patient is awake with no obvious life-threats, begin a more in-depth assessment of the patient's mentation (alertness and orientation to surroundings).

- Person: Does the patient know his or her name?
- Place: Does the patient know where he or she is?
- Time: Does the patient know the year, month, and approximate date and time?
- Event: Can the patient describe the current MOI or NOI?

D. ABC (or CAB if patient unresponsive or major bleeding)

> ➤ *Remember:* ABC vs. CAB: You **must** assess LOC to determine if your primary assessment will follow the Airway, Breathing, Circulation (ABC) approach or the Circulation, Airway, Breathing (CAB) approach. Unconscious or severe bleeding = CAB. Everyone else = ABC. *This is a critical concept!*

  1. Clarifying ABC vs. CAB

      i. Responsive patients do **not** need CPR. Use ABC approach.

      ii. Unconscious patients **may** need CPR. Use CAB approach.

      iii. Life-threatening external bleeding **must** be controlled immediately. Use CAB approach.

  2. Airway

      i. The patient's LOC is a key factor in determining what airway interventions are needed. Do **not** assume that patients with a decreased LOC are able to adequately protect their own airway.

      ii. Three key steps in airway management (as indicated):

- Manual
  - Head-tilt, chin-lift
  - Jaw thrust

- Suction
  - — Suction upper airway as needed
- Mechanical
  - — Basic life support: Oropharyngeal airway (unresponsive patients **only**), nasopharyngeal airway (decreased LOC).
  - — ALS: Supraglottic airway, intubation, etc.

3. Breathing
   i. Support ventilations and provide supplemental oxygen as indicated.
      - Assess for signs of criticality (LOC, rate, tidal volume, SpO_2, etc.).
      - Maintain SpO_2 of 94%–99%.
      - Manage flail chest (with PPV) and sucking chest wounds (with occlusive dressing) as indicated.
      - If BVM ventilation is indicated, do **not** hyperventilate. Maintain SpO_2 of 94%–99% and $ETCO_2$ of 35–45 mmHg.

4. Circulation
   i. Bleeding
      - Manage life-threatening bleeding immediately.
        - — Direct pressure
        - — Tourniquet
        - — Hemostatic agents or junctional tourniquet as indicated
      - See Bleeding and Shock chapter for additional information.
   ii. Pulse
      - CPR as indicated.
      - Remember: CPR is indicated for pulseless patients and unresponsive pediatric patients with a pulse less than 60 beats/min.
   iii. Skin (color, temperature, moisture)
      - Assess for signs of hypoxia, e.g., cyanosis.

- Assess for signs of shock, e.g., pale (pallor), cool, clammy.
- Assess for signs of infection, e.g., jaundice, rash.
- Pediatric considerations, e.g., capillary refill, mottling, marbling.

> *Remember:* The rapid scan is intended specifically to identify any remaining life-threatening conditions and should **not** take longer than about 90 seconds.

5. Rapid scan (rapid secondary)
    i. The rapid scan is a rapid head-to-toe assessment used specifically to identify any remaining life-threatening conditions not already managed. Examples: signs of internal bleeding, pelvic fracture, femur fracture, traumatic brain injury (TBI).
    ii. Indicated for all unresponsive patients (medical or trauma), significant trauma patients, or any patient you suspect may have additional life-threatening conditions.
    iii. Do **not** spend time on non-life-threatening conditions during the rapid scan.
    iv. Inspect (look), palpate (touch), and auscultate (listen) for life threats.
    v. Remember to assess the posterior for any life-threatening conditions if not done during the primary assessment.

6. Transport priority
    i. Form your field impression, e.g., sick or not sick? Stable or unstable?
    ii. Do **not** delay transport of a high-priority patient to manage non-life-threatening conditions.
    iii. A few significant MOIs indicating probable need for high-priority transport to an appropriate trauma center:
        - Falls over 20 feet in adults or over 10 feet in children.
        - Any fall leading to a traumatic loss of consciousness.
        - Motor vehicle collisions (MVC) with more than 12 inches of intrusion into occupant space.
        - MVC with ejection.

- ➤ Death of another occupant in same vehicle.
- ➤ Pedestrian or cyclist struck by vehicle.
- ➤ Motorcycle accident over 20 mph.
- ➤ *Note:* Two or more significant MOIs significantly risk likelihood of life-threatening injury.

V. PATIENT HISTORY

A. For most conscious medical patients, the most important information usually comes from the patient history.

B. Interpersonal communication
   1. **Do this:**
      i. Introduce yourself and get patient's name (and use it).
      ii. Make eye contact.
      iii. Position yourself at same or lower level.
      iv. Be honest.
      v. Use appropriate language, terminology that patient can understand.
      vi. Allow patient time to answer.
   2. **Don't** do this:
      i. Provide false assurance or lie.
      ii. Give advice.
      iii. Act authoritarian.
      iv. Use professional jargon.
      v. Use leading or biased questions.
      vi. Talk too much or interrupt.
      vii. Ask "why" questions.

C. SAMPLE history
   1. **Signs and symptoms**
   2. **Allergies**

3. Medications
4. Past history
5. Last oral intake
6. Events leading to incident

D. OPQRST
1. **Onset**
2. **Provocation**
3. **Quality**
4. **Radiation**
5. **Severity**
6. **Time**

E. PASTE assessment for dyspnea (an alternative to OPQRST)
1. **P:** Provoking factors
2. **A:** Associated pain
3. **S:** Sputum
4. **T:** Time of onset and temperature
5. **E:** Exacerbation, exercise

F. Associated symptoms and pertinent negatives
1. Associated symptoms: Other symptoms associated with the chief complaint.
    i. **Example:** Chief complaint is chest pain, but patient also complains of dyspnea.
2. Pertinent negatives: Potential associated symptoms that are NOT present.
    i. Example: Trauma patient denies neck pain.

> *Remember:* All life-threatening conditions should be managed **before** starting the secondary assessment. Do **not** delay transport of a high-priority patient to complete a secondary assessment.

Patient Assessment

VI. SECONDARY ASSESSMENT

A. The four assessment techniques
   1. Inspection: Observe.
   2. Palpation: Touch.
   3. Auscultation: Listen.
   4. Percussion: Not frequently used prehospital.

B. Secondary assessment tips
   1. The secondary assessment should **not** delay transport of a high-priority patient.
   2. The secondary assessment is designed to identify any remaining conditions or injuries.
   3. The secondary assessment can be a detailed head-to-toe assessment or a focused assessment that assesses only relevant areas.
      i. Indications for a head-to-toe secondary assessment include:
         ➤ Unresponsive or otherwise unable to provide feedback.
         ➤ Multisystem trauma.
         ➤ High-priority transport.
      ii. Indications for a focused secondary assessment include conscious patients with a specific, isolated chief complaint (medical or trauma).

   ➤ *Remember:* Jugular vein distention (JVD) is common in supine patients. JVD in seated patients may be an indication of various medical problems (right heart failure, cardiac tamponade, tension pneumothorax, pulmonary embolism). **Always** assess lung sounds and consider causes for any patient with abnormal JVD.

C. Body systems assessment
   1. HEENT: head, eyes, ears, nose, throat
   2. Chest and lungs
   3. Abdomen (GI/GU)

Chapter 4

    4. Musculoskeletal

    5. Neurological

    6. Hematologic

    7. Endocrine

    8. Psychiatric

D. Assess for DCAP-BLS-TIC (formerly DCAP-BTLS) for trauma and unresponsive patients).

    1. Inspect for (injuries that can be seen):
        i. **D**eformities.
        ii. **C**ontusions.
        iii. **A**brasions.
        iv. **P**enetrating injuries and paradoxical motion.
        v. **B**urns.
        vi. **L**acerations.
        vii. **S**welling.

    2. Palpate for (injuries that must be felt):
        i. **T**enderness.
        ii. **I**nstability.
        iii. **C**repitus.

E. Baseline vitals

    1. Respirations

    2. Pulse

    3. Blood pressure (BP)

    4. Temperature

    5. Skin

    6. Pupils

    7. Pulse oximetry, $ETCO_2$ (as indicated)

    8. Blood glucose (as indicated)

Patient Assessment

Advanced Medical Assessment						
X:	Manage Life-threatening bleeding					
Airway:		S:		O:		P:
Breathing:		A:		P:		A:
Circulation:		M:		Q:		S:
Disability:		P:		R:		T:
Expose/Environ:		L:		S:		E:
Name:	Age:		E:		T:	
Chief Complaint:			R:		I:	
Resp:	Differential Diagnosis: Likely ↓ Unlikely Cardiac | Resp | Endo/Met Neuro | Infection | Shock| GI/GU	Antidepressants • Amitriptyline (Elavil) • Amoxapine (Asendin) • Aripiprazole (Abilify) • Bupropion (Wellbutrin) • Citalopram (Celexa) • Duloxetine (Cymbalta) • Escitalopram (Lexapro) • Fluoxetine (Prozac) • Imipramine (Tofranil) • Isocarboxazid (Marplan) • Nortriptyline (Pamelor) • Paroxetine (Paxil) • Quetiapine (Seroquel) • Selegiline (Emsam) • Sertraline (Zoloft) • Tranylcypromine (Parnate) • Trazodone (Dysyrel) • Venlafaxine (Effexor)			Beta blockers • Atenolol (Tenormin) • Metoprolol (Lopressor) • Propranolol (Inderal) • Labetalol **Blood thinners** • Apixaban (Eliquis) • Dabigatran (Pradaxa) • Edoxaban (Savaysa) • Enoxaparin (Lovenox) • Heparin • Rivaroxaban (Xarelto) • Warfarin (Jantoven) **ED meds** • Avanafil (Stendra) • Sildenafil (Viagra) • Tadalafil (Cialis) • Vardenafil (Levitra)	
Pulse:						
BP:						
SPO₂:						
ETCO₂:						
BG:						
Lungs:						
ECG:						
12 Lead:						
Physical:				Glasgow Coma Scale			

EYES:	Open spontaneously	4
	To verbal stimulus	3
	To painful stimulus	2
	No response	1
MOTOR:	Obeys verbal	6
	Localizes pain	5
	Semi-purposeful	4
	Decorticate	3
	Decerebrate	2
	No response	1
VERBAL:	Oriented	5
	Disoriented	4
	Inappropriate words	3
	Incomprehensible	2
	No response	2
Total:	3-15	

Stridor
• High-pitched
• Upper airway to trachea
• Usually inspiratory
• FBAO
• Croup
• Burns/chemicals
• Anaphylaxis
• Epiglottitis

Wheezes
• High-pitched
• Lower airway
• Usually expiratory
• Asthma
• Anaphylaxis
• COPD

Rales/Crackles
• Wet/fluid
• Lower airway (alveoli)
• Usually inspiratory
• Pulmonary edema

Rhonchi
• Course/low-pitched
• Lower airway
• Usually expiratory
• Mucus
• Infection
• Bronchitis
• Cystic fibrosis

AEIOUTIPS

Life Threat | Critical | Non-Emergent

Treatment:	Reassessment:

Stroke | Sepsis | Trauma | STEMI

Document developed by the Contra Costa College Paramedic Program, class 23-1

Figure 4-1: Sample Advanced Medical Assessment

|79

Chapter 4

 VII. REASSESSMENT

   A. Reassessment tips

   1. The purpose of the reassessment phase is to monitor for changes in the patient's condition.

   2. Reassess stable patients every 15 minute and unstable patients every 5 minutes.

   3. Continue reassessment until transfer of care or until patient's condition requires repeat of the primary assessment.

   B. Components of reassessment

   1. Reassess LOC.

   2. Reassess ABCs.

   3. Reassess chief complaint.

   4. Reassess interventions.

   5. Reassess vitals.

 VIII. PRINCIPLES OF ALS MANAGEMENT

   A. General management of ALS patients

   1. Manage ABCs as indicated.

   2. Complete thorough patient assessment as indicated.

   3. Supplemental oxygen and PPV as indicated.

      i. *Note:* Always administer supplemental oxygen to patients with suspected hypoxia, shock, or TBI.

      ii. To avoid hyperoxia in stable patients, titrate oxygen therapy to an SpO_2 of 94%–99%.

   4. Monitor vitals, ECG, SpO_2, $ETCO_2$ as indicated.

   5. Assess blood glucose as indicated.

   6. IV access and fluid resuscitation (NaCL or lactated Ringer's) as indicated.

   7. Transport as indicated.

B. *Note:* In the following chapters, the above will simply be referred to as "general management of ALS patients."

C. See appropriate chapters for specific interventions based on conditions, injuries, or illnesses.

  IX. PEDIATRIC ASSESSMENT TIPS

A. Infants (up to 1 year)
  1. Should be alert, engaged with environment.
  2. Arms and legs should move bilaterally.
  3. Should recognize parents (over 2 months of age).
  4. Normal vitals:
     i. Respirations: 30–60.
     ii. Heart rate: 100–180.
     iii. Systolic BP: at least 70 to about 104.

B. Toddlers (1–3 years)
  1. Should be walking by 18 months.
  2. Often disagreeable.
  3. Most trusting of parents/guardians.
  4. May not want to be touched.
  5. Focus on vital areas (based on complaint) first.
  6. Normal vitals:
     i. Respirations: 24–40.
     ii. Heart rate: 80–110.
     iii. Systolic BP: about 80 + 2(age in years).

C. Preschoolers (3–6 years)
  1. Often distrustful of strangers.
  2. May fear sight of blood, injury.
  3. Answer questions honestly.

4. Normal vitals
    i. Respirations: 22–34.
    ii. Heart rate: 70–110.
    iii. Systolic BP: about 80 + 2(age in years).

D. School-age (6–12 years)
   1. Often cooperative if they trust you.
   2. Often seek control.
   3. Offer choices.
   4. May be modest, resist physical examination.
   5. Normal vitals:
       i. Respirations: 18–30.
       ii. Heart rate: 65–110.
       iii. Systolic BP: about 80 + 2(age in years).

E. Adolescents (13–18 years)
   1. Treat similar to adults.
   2. Can be extremely modest.
   3. Consider same-sex provider if possible.
   4. Normal vitals:
       i. Respirations: 12–26.
       ii. Heart rate: 60–90.
       iii. Systolic BP: 110–130.

X. SUMMARY OF PATIENT ASSESSMENT

A. Scene size-up
   1. Scene safety, standard precautions
   2. No. of patients, additional resources
   3. Consider MOI or NOI, spinal precautions

B. Primary assessment

  1. ABCs or CAB (if unresponsive)
  2. Rapid scan as indicated
  3. Determine transport priority

C. Patient history (may come before or after secondary assessment)

  1. SAMPLE

D. Secondary assessment

  1. Detailed assessment or focused assessment (as indicated)

E. Reassessment

  1. Reassess patient's chief complaint, vitals, interventions, etc.

REVIEW QUESTIONS
(Answers on pg. 413.)

1. After the scene size-up, what precedes all other components of patient assessment?

   A. reassessment
   B. focused exam
   C. vital signs
   D. primary assessment

2. What is the purpose of the primary assessment?

   A. identify and manage all injuries or conditions
   B. identify and manage life-threatening injuries or conditions
   C. obtain a complete set of vital signs
   D. determine MOI or history of present illness (HPI)

Chapter 4

3. How will you determine if the ABC or the CAB approach to the primary assessment is indicated?

    A. the patient's LOC
    B. the MOI or HPI
    C. the chief complaint
    D. the baseline vital signs

4. Your pediatric patient is unresponsive and has a pulse of 50 beats per minute. You should immediately:

    A. administer atropine.
    B. check the blood glucose.
    C. provide supplemental oxygen.
    D. begin CPR.

5. Which of the following statements regarding JVD is most accurate?

    A. JVD should be assessed while the patient is in the Fowler or semi-Fowler position.
    B. JVD should be assessed while the patient is supine.
    C. JVD should be assessed only in unresponsive patients.
    D. JVD should be assessed during the scene size-up.

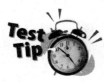

Be sure to know the "general management of ALS patients" referred to throughout the book. These are the foundational assessments and interventions for paramedics.

Patient Monitoring Technology

Chapter 5

I. TERMS TO KNOW

A. **Capnography:** Measure or monitoring of exhaled CO_2.

B. **Infarct:** Area of necrosis, or death.

C. **Pulse CO-oximetry (SpCO):** Noninvasive measurement of carbon monoxide saturation of hemoglobin.

D. **Pulse oximetry (SpO$_2$):** Noninvasive measurement of oxygen saturation of hemoglobin.

E. **SpMet:** Noninvasive measurement of methemoglobin.

II. PATIENT MONITORING TECH USED IN PREHOSPITAL

A. ECG monitoring and 12-lead ECG

B. Pulse oximetry

C. Pulse CO-oximetry

D. Capnography

E. Methemoglobin monitoring

F. Total hemoglobin monitoring

G. Glucometry

85

Chapter 5

III. ECG MONITORING

A. Bipolar leads
1. Lead I: Negative electrode right arm and positive electrode left arm.
2. Lead II: Negative electrode right arm and positive electrode left leg.
3. Lead III: Negative electrode left arm and positive electrode left leg.

B. Limitations
1. Provides no information regarding mechanical cardiac function.
2. Nondiagnostic for myocardial infarction (MI).

C. Basic ECG rhythms to know
1. Sinus: Normal sinus rhythm, sinus bradycardia, sinus tachycardia.
2. Atrial: Supraventricular tachycardia, atrial flutter, atrial fibrillation.
3. Junctional: Junctional escape rhythm, accelerated junctional rhythm, junctional tachycardia.
4. Ventricular: Ventricular escape rhythm, accelerated ventricular rhythm, ventricular tachycardia, ventricular fibrillation, asystole.
5. AV blocks: First-degree, second-degree type I, second-degree type II, third-degree.
6. Cardiac arrest rhythms: Asystole, ventricular fibrillation, pulseless ventricular tachycardia, pulseless electrical activity.

IV. 12-LEAD ECG

A. Prehospital indications
1. Suspected acute coronary syndrome/MI
    i. Chest pain
    ii. Dyspnea
    iii. Diaphoresis
    iv. Palpitations
    v. Anxiety

2. Possible signs and symptoms of abnormal MI presentation
    i. Syncope
    ii. Epigastric pain
    iii. Pulmonary edema
    iv. Weakness

B. Advantages
    1. Diagnostic for myocardial ischemia, injury, infarct.
    2. Can provide earlier recognition and management of ST-segment elevation myocardial infarction (STEMI).
    3. Indicated for patients with any indication of possible cardiac problem.
    4. Identification of high-risk ECG findings, such as QT prolongation.
    5. Use of right-sided leads not necessary if STEMI has been identified.

C. Limitations
    1. Provides no information regarding mechanical cardiac function.
    2. Standard 12-lead provides limited information about right ventricle and posterior left ventricle.

D. Zones of myocardial damage
    1. Ischemia
        i. Myocardium receiving inadequate oxygen (reversible condition).
        ii. ECG: ST depression, inverted T waves, or peaked T waves.
            ➤ *Note:* ST depression must be at least one small box below baseline.
    2. Injury
        i. Myocardial damage due to ischemia (potentially reversible condition).
        ii. ECG: ST elevation.
            ➤ *Note:* ST elevation must be at least 1 mm in two or more continuous leads.

Chapter 5

3. Infarction
    i. Myocardial death (irreversible condition).
    ii. ECG: Significant (pathological) Q wave.
        ➤ *Note:* Pathological Q wave must be at least 1 mm (0.04 seconds) wide or deeper than one-third the R wave (in same lead).

E. Lead placement (12-lead)

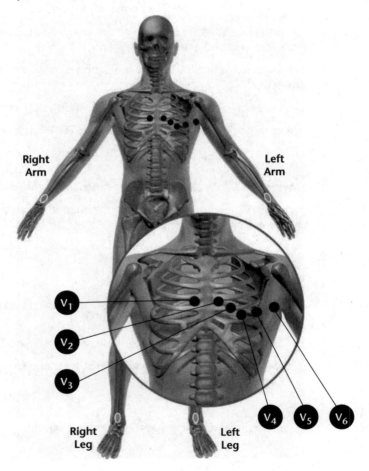

Patient Monitoring Technology

Electrode	Placement Area
V_1	Fourth intercostal space to the right of the sternum.
V_2	Fourth intercostal space to the left of the sternum.
V_3	Directly between leads V_2 and V_4.
V_4	Fifth intercostal space at midclavicular line.
V_5	Level with V_4 at left anterior axillary line.
V_6	Level with V_5 at the midaxillary line. (Directly under the midpoint of the armpit)

https://www.numed.co.uk/news/12-lead-ecg-lead-placement-guide>

1. Bipolar leads: I, II, III
2. Unipolar (augmented) leads: aVR, aVL, aVF
3. Chest (precordial) leads: V_1–V_6
    i. V_1: Fourth intercostal space, right of sternum
    ii. V_2: Fourth intercostal space, left of sternum
    iii. V_3: Between V_2 and V_4
    iv. V_4: Fifth intercostal space, midclavicular
    v. V_5: Anterior axillary line, level with V_4
    vi. V_6: Midaxillary line, level with V_4 (just under mid armpit)
4. Lead groupings ("I See All Leads" mnemonic)
    i. Inferior leads: Leads II, III, aVF
        ➤ *Note:* Inferior MI doesn't contraindicate use of nitroglycerin; however, use caution when blood pressure is marginal.
        ➤ Consider risk vs. benefit of nitroglycerin and opiate analgesics.
        ➤ Be prepared to administer fluid bolus and vasopressor medications for hypotension.
    ii. Septal leads: V_1, V_2
    iii. Anterior leads: V_3, V_4
    iv. Lateral leads: Lead I, aVL, V_5, V_6

V. PULSE OXIMETRY (SpO$_2$)

A. Uses
1. Noninvasive and indirect method of monitoring oxygen saturation of hemoglobin (SpO$_2$).
   i. *Tip:* SpO$_2$ readings are a percentage; therefore max value is 100.
   ii. *Tip:* SaO$_2$ (unlike SpO$_2$) is a direct and invasive measurement (arterial blood gas). So easy to confuse these, but we medics use SpO$_2$!
2. Monitoring of pulse rate
   i. *Tip:* Unlike an ECG, the SpO$_2$ monitor **can** provide info about mechanical cardiac function.
   ii. Most SpO$_2$ devices provide visual and auditory monitoring of pulse (that annoying, but sometimes helpful "BEEP"). Ex: Auditory monitoring of pulse for possible bradycardia in pediatric patients or newborns.
   iii. *Tip:* SpO$_2$ could be useful in assessing circulation distal to a suspected orthopedic fracture or for identifying inapparent hypoxia in patients with long bone fractures.

B. SpO$_2$ values
1. Normal: 94%–100%.
2. Below 94%: Suspect hypoxia, shock, or respiratory compromise.
3. Below 90%: Aggressive airway management, ventilatory support, and high-flow oxygen indicated.
4. *Note:* Patients with chronic obstructive pulmonary disease may routinely have SpO$_2$ readings as low as 85%.
5. Indications
   i. Dyspnea or other indications of respiratory compromise
   ii. Suspected hypoxia
   iii. Altered level of consciousness (LOC)
   iv. Suspected shock, multisystem trauma
   v. Traumatic brain injury (TBI)
   vi. Suspected MI or stroke

Patient Monitoring Technology

vii. Patients receiving analgesics or sedation medications

viii. Any patient receiving supplemental oxygen or positive pressure ventilation (PPV)

ix. Possible identification of inapparent hypoxia after long bone fractures

x. Use to maintain patient's SpO_2 at 94%–99% or above

xi. *Note:* Excessive oxygen administration (hyperoxia) can have harmful effects, e.g., coronary and cerebral artery vasoconstriction. Titrate to 94%–99% instead of 100% to reduce risk of complications.

6. Limitations

   i. Inaccurate readings possible due to:
   - Hypoperfusion (Example: hemorrhage, dehydration, hypothermia).
   - Anemia (anemic patients can have an SpO_2 of 100%, despite being dangerously anemic).
   - CO poisoning (device only reads percentage on bound hemoglobin, not what is bound to that hemoglobin, e.g., O_2 vs. CO).
   - Methemoglobinemia/cyanide poisoning.
   - Sunlight.
   - Nail polish.
   - Poor probe placement, movement.

   ii. Does not indicate total respiratory or circulatory sufficiency; must be used with other assessments, physical exam, etc.

   iii. There can be a delay in desaturation readings (not an immediate, real-time indicator of patient's condition).

VI. CAPNOGRAPHY

A. $ETCO_2$ provides real-time information regarding cellular metabolism, circulation, and ventilation.

1. *Note:* Capnography and capnometry are often used synonymously; however, capnography indicates continuous monitoring (numerical or waveform), while capnometry indicates analysis without continuous monitoring.

Chapter 5

B. ETCO$_2$ values
  1. Normal ETCO$_2$: 35–45 mmHg
  2. Elevated ETCO$_2$ (greater than 45 mmHg) = acidosis
      i. Increase rate of PPV (for patients being ventilated).
  3. Decreased ETCO$_2$ (below 35 mmHg) = hyperventilation
      i. Decrease rate of PPV (the patient is likely being hyperventilated).

C. Capnography devices
  1. Colorimetric devices
      i. Disposable, color-changing ETCO$_2$ detector.
      ii. Used to help verify endotracheal tube (ETT) placement or indicate ETT displacement (**not** a substitute for continuous waveform capnography).
      iii. Limitations are extensive, such as no numerical value and no waveform.
  2. Electronic capnography can provide a numerical value or a numerical value and a waveform.

D. Indications and advantages of continuous ETCO$_2$ monitoring
  1. Continuous ETT monitoring.
  2. Monitor effectiveness of CPR.
  3. Monitor adequacy of ventilations.
  4. Improved management of patients with increased intracranial pressure, particularly during PPV.
  5. Excessive condensation in ETCO$_2$ probe or device can disrupt monitoring.
  6. *Note:* Target ventilations of patients with TBI to an SpO$_2$ of 94%–99% and an ETCO$_2$ of 40 mmHg.

VII. PULSE CO-OXIMETRY (SpCO)

A. Carbon monoxide (CO) binds to hemoglobin 200 times stronger than oxygen does, causing carboxyhemoglobin (a common toxicologic emergency).

Patient Monitoring Technology

   B. Firefighters at increased risk of chronic and acute exposure to CO.

   C. SpCO provides rapid, noninvasive detection of CO poisoning. SpCO devices also provide SpO_2 and pulse rate data.

   D. SpCO values and interventions
      1. 0%–3%: Normal.
      2. 3%–12%: Administer high-flow oxygen and transport if symptomatic, or known exposure to CO.
      3. Above 12%: Administer high-flow oxygen and transport.
      4. *Note:* Any symptomatic patient with known CO exposure should be transported, regardless of SpCO reading.
      5. *Note:* At least mild symptoms are present once carboxyhemoglobin reaches about 15%.
      6. *Note:* Consider hyperbaric chamber for patients with excessively high SpCO, especially pediatric patients and pregnant females.

   E. Indications
      1. Known or suspected exposure to CO
      2. Persistent hypoxia despite oxygen therapy
      3. Altered LOC of unknown etiology

   F. Limitations
      1. Similar to SpO_2 devices
      2. *Note:* Elevated SpMet levels in the blood can result in falsely elevated SpCO reading.

VIII. METHEMOGLOBINEMIA MONITORING (SpMet)

   A. High levels of methemoglobin (MetHb) disrupt the hemoglobin's ability to transport and deliver oxygen to the cells, causing hypoxia.

   B. Some SpCO monitors can measure MetHb levels (measured as SpMet).

Chapter 5

    C. SpMet values

        1. 1%–3% SpMet: Normal.

        2. 3%–15% SpMet: Ashen or cyanotic skin possible.

        3. 15%–20% SpMet: Cyanosis.

        4. 25%–50% SpMet: Headache, dyspnea, altered LOC.

        5. 50%–70% SpMet: Altered or decreased LOC.

        6. 70% SpMet or above: Fatal.

    D. Indications

        1. Cyanosis unresolved by oxygen therapy

        2. Patients receiving intravenous nitrates, lidocaine, nitric oxide.

        3. Suspected cyanide exposure

        4. Any patient with elevated SpCO levels

    E. Limitations

        1. Similar to SpO_2 and SpCO devices.

IX. TOTAL HEMOGLOBIN MONITORING

    A. Some SpCO monitors can measure total hemoglobin concentrations (measured as SpHb) and help identify patients with dehydration or hemorrhage.

    B. Normal hemoglobin (Hb) values are age-dependent.

        1. Newborns – 2 weeks: 14.5–24.5 g/dL

        2. Infants up to 8 weeks: 12.5–20.5 g/dL

        3. Infants up to 6 months: 10.7–17.3 g/dL

        4. Infants up to 1 year: 9.9–14.5 g/dL

        5. Children up to 6 years: 9.5–14.1 g/dL

        6. Adult males: 14–17.4 g/dL

        7. Adult females: 12–16 g/dL

Patient Monitoring Technology

- C. Abnormal SpHb (remember, SpHb is the indirect, noninvasive measure of Hb levels)
    1. High SpHb: Suspect dehydration (hemoconcentration due to low plasma).
    2. Low SpHb: Suspect hemorrhage, anemia.
- D. Indications for SpHb monitoring
    1. Suspected dehydration or hemorrhage
    2. Suspected hypoperfusion (shock)

X. GLUCOMETRY

- A. Indications
    1. Known or suspected diabetic history
    2. Altered or decreased LOC
    3. Seizures
    4. Stroke
    5. Pregnancy
    6. Suspected alcohol abuse
    7. Suspected overdose
    8. Any time you have any reason to even remotely suspect an abnormal blood glucose level (it's fast, easy, minimally invasive)
- B. Blood glucose values
    1. Ideally, blood glucose levels are tested after fasting. A fasting blood glucose level of 99 mg/dL or less is considered normal. A fasting blood glucose of 100 mg/dL or higher indicates possible prediabetes or diabetes.
    2. Nonfasting blood glucose levels
        i. Normal levels:
            - Normal (adult, nondiabetic): About 70–120 mg/dL
            - Normal (adult, diabetic): About 100–180 mg/dL
            - Normal (newborn): Above 40 mg/dL

ii. A blood glucose level of 140 mg/dL is not unusual just after eating.

iii. A blood glucose level over 200 mg/dL indicates diabetes.

3. Continuous glucose monitoring and automated insulin delivery is now possible for diabetics using an insulin pump with a tiny sensor placed under the skin (usually on the abdomen or arm). The sensor tests glucose levels every few minutes and transmits the data to a monitor, phone, etc.

4. A1C blood glucose testing averages blood sugar levels over several months. The results are reported as a percentage. A normal A1C level is below 5.7%. Above 5.7% indicates chronic hyperglycemia.

5. Estimated average glucose (eAG) provides average blood glucose levels for past 6–90 days. Can be reported in mg/dL or millimoles per liter (mmol/L).

6. The international standard of measuring blood glucose is mmol/L; 1 mmol/L = 18 mg/dL.

REVIEW QUESTIONS
(Answers on pg. 414.)

1. Which of the following are considered bipolar leads?

   A. I, II, III

   B. aVR, aVL, aVF

   C. V_1–V_6

   D. All leads are bipolar leads.

2. Which of the following are collectively considered the inferior view lead grouping?

   A. V_1, V_2

   B. V_3, V_4

   C. II, III, aVF

   D. I, aVL, V_5, V_6

3. Bag-valve-mask ventilations of a TBI patient should be targeted to:
   A. SpO$_2$ of at least 94% and an ETCO$_2$ of 40 mmHg.
   B. SpO$_2$ of at least 90% and an ETCO$_2$ of 30 mmHg.
   C. SpO$_2$ of 100% and an ETCO$_2$ of at least 45 mmHg.
   D. SpO$_2$ of at least 85% and an ETCO$_2$ of at least 50 mmHg.

4. Which of the following is a normal nonfasting blood glucose level?
   A. 99 mg/dL or less
   B. 100–180 mg/dL
   C. 70–120 mg/dL
   D. 200 mg/dL or above

5. Your adult female patient has an SpHb of 20 g/dL. This indicates:
   A. a normal SpHb level for an adult female.
   B. probable hemorrhage.
   C. probable anemia.
   D. probable dehydration.

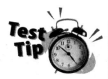

The certification exam places a strong emphasis on anatomy, physiology, pathophysiology, and terminology. Be sure to review the "Terms to Know" sections in the book and the "Anatomy & Physiology Review" online at www.rea.com/paramedic.

Bleeding and Shock

Chapter 6

I. TERMS TO KNOW

A. **Anaphylactic shock:** Life-threating allergic reaction; aka anaphylaxis.

B. **Beck's triad:** Jugluar vein distention, muffled heart tones, and hypotension/narrowing pulse pressure. Collectively, they indicated cardiac tamponade (a form of obstructive shock).

C. **Cardiac tamponade:** Compression of the heart due to an accumulation of fluid in the pericardial sac (aka pericardial tamponade).

D. **Compensated shock:** Early shock where the body still maintains adequate perfusion.

E. **Cullen's sign:** Periumbilical bruising.

F. **Decompensated shock:** Later shock where the body can no longer maintain adequate perfusion.

G. **Distributive shock:** Includes neurogenic shock, anaphylactic shock, and septic shock.

H. **Grey Turner's sign:** Bruising of the flanks. Possible indication of retroperitoneal hemorrhage.

I. **Hematemesis:** Vomiting blood.

J. **Hematochezia:** Bloody stool.

K. **Hemorrhage:** Bleeding.

L. **Irreversible shock:** Stage of shock leading to inevitable death.

M. **Mean arterial pressure (MAP):** DBP + 1/3 (SBP − DBP) or alternate calculation: $\frac{2(DBP) + SBP}{3}$.

N. **Melena:** Dark stool.

O. **Multiple organ dysfunction syndrome:** Progressive failure of at least two organ systems.

P. **Neurogenic shock:** Shock due to neurologic injury leading to loss of sympathetic tone.

Q. **Obstructive shock:** Includes cardiac tamponade, tension pneumothorax, and pulmonary embolism.

R. **Septic shock:** Shock due to infection; aka sepsis.

S. **Urticaria:** Hives.

> ➤ *Remember:* External bleeding is the **single most preventable cause of traumatic death**; therefore, it **must** be managed quickly and aggressively.

II. BLEEDING

A. Types of bleeding
  1. External
     i. *Note:* Remember to expose any patient with suspected bleeding.
     ii. Check for bleeding from places that may not be obvious, e.g., posterior, axillary regions.
  2. Internal
     i. A single femur fracture, pelvic fracture, or multiple long bone fractures can lead to hemorrhagic shock.
     ii. Signs of internal hemorrhage
        ➤ Bruising
        ➤ Hematoma
        ➤ Hematemesis (vomiting blood)

- Coffee ground–like emesis
- Bloody stool (hematochezia)
- Dark, tarry stool (melena)
- Abdominal distention or rigidity
- Suspected femur or pelvic fracture
- Grey Turner's sign
- Signs and symptoms of shock

B. Sources of bleeding
   1. Arterial bleeding: Spurting, bright red blood.
   2. Venous bleeding: Steady flowing, dark red.
   3. Capillary bleeding: Slow, oozing dark red blood.

> *Remember:* There are **no** widely accepted indications for use of medical anti-shock trousers (MAST)/pneumatic anti shock garment (PASG) according to the American College of Surgeons and the American College of Emergency Physicians.

C. Management of bleeding
   1. External bleeding
      i. First method: **Direct pressure**
         - Consider hemostatic dressings and/or wound packing per local protocol.
      ii. Second method: **Tourniquet**
         - Use commercial tourniquet if available and per local protocol.
         - Can use blood pressure (BP) cuff as last resort (monitor for leaks).
         - Always place tourniquet proximal to injury (2"–3").
         - Apply enough pressure to control bleeding.
         - Do not apply directly over joint.
         - Write "TK" and time applied on tape and secure to patient's forehead and notify transfer of care personnel.

- If bleeding is in a location that will not allow use of a traditional tourniquet, consider hemostatic dressing or junctional tourniquet (Example: SAM Junctional Tourniquet, Combat Ready Clamp) per local protocol.
- Risk of permanent tissue damage less than previously thought if used for under 2 hours.
- Use of arterial pressure points is **no longer recommended**.

iii. Special situations
- Wound packing or a junctional tourniquet are indicated for groin/axillary ("junctional") injury with significant bleeding not controllable with direct pressure or regular tourniquet.
- Epistaxis (nosebleed)
  — Consider cause, e.g., trauma, hypertension.
  — Have patient lean forward, avoid swallowing blood.
  — Pinch nostrils below bridge of nose for at least 10 minutes.
- Bleeding from nose or ears following head injury
  — Consider possibility of skull fracture.
  — Apply loose dressing, but do not apply direct pressure.
- Additional information (e.g., impaled objects and open neck wounds): See chapter on Soft Tissue and Orthopedic Injuries.

2. Suspected internal bleeding
  i. General management of advanced life support patients.
  ii. Treat for shock.
  iii. Consider pelvic binder for suspected pelvic fracture.
  iv. Rapid transport.

III. SHOCK

A. Shock (aka hypoperfusion) is any condition causing inadequate tissue perfusion due to reduced cardiac output.

B. Three primary causes of shock (aka the "Perfusion Triangle")

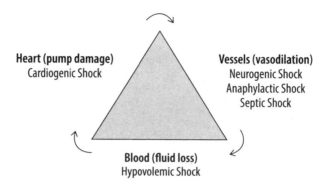

Figure 6-1: Perfusion Triangle

1. Pump (cardiac) problem
    i. Example: cardiogenic shock
2. Pipes (vasodilation) problem
    i. Example: anaphylactic shock
3. Fluid (hypovolemic) problem
    i. Example: hemorrhagic shock

C. Impaired oxygenation and glucose

1. All causes of shock lead to impaired oxygenation due to anaerobic (without oxygen) metabolic function.
2. Anaerobic metabolism creates little energy and increased acidosis.
3. Shock also causes impaired glucose delivery to cells, increasing risk of organ failure.

IV. CATEGORIES (STAGES) OF SHOCK

A. Compensated shock

1. The body's defense mechanisms are compensating for the decrease in cardiac output.

Chapter 6

2. Compensatory mechanisms
   i. Increased heart rate and cardiac force of contraction
   ii. Increased vasoconstriction
   iii. Reduced urinary output to maintain intravascular volume

> **Remember:** The telltale characteristic of decompensated shock is a falling BP leading to hypotension. **Do not** wait for hypotension to identify decompensated shock.

B. Decompensated (progressive) shock
   1. The body's defense mechanisms are no longer able to compensate for the decrease in cardiac output.
   2. Falling or low BP are hallmark signs of decompensated shock.
   3. Importance of mean arterial pressure (MAP)
      i. MAP = DBP + 1/3 (SBP − DBP).
      ii. Normal MAP is 70–100. A MAP of at least 60 is needed to perfuse vital organs.

C. Irreversible shock
   1. Irrecoverable shock leading to inevitable death

> **Remember:** Patients in neurogenic shock will **not** likely present with tachycardia or pale, cool, clammy skin (below the level of injury). Neurogenic shock patients **will** be hypotensive.

V. CLASSIFICATION (TYPES) OF SHOCK

A. Older classification system
   1. Cardiogenic shock (pump problem)
   2. Hypovolemic shock (fluid problem)
   3. Neurogenic shock (vasodilation problem)
   4. Anaphylactic shock (vasodilation/permeability problem)

5. Septic shock (vasodilation/permeability problem)

> **Remember:** The classic triad of findings for cardiac tamponade (a form of obstructive shock) is called Beck's triad and includes jugular vein distention, muffled heart tones, and hypotension.

B. Newer classification system
   1. Cardiogenic shock
   2. Hypovolemic shock
   3. Obstructive shock
      i. Pulmonary embolism
      ii. Cardiac tamponade
      iii. Tension pneumothorax

> **Remember:** "Relative" hypovolemia means there is not enough blood volume relative to the size of the vascular space. Distributive shock can cause massive systemic vasodilation, resulting in relative hypovolemia and hypotension.

   4. Distributive shock (aka "warm" shock)
      i. Neurogenic shock
      ii. Anaphylactic shock
      iii. Septic shock

VI. SIGNS, SYMPTOMS, AND MANAGEMENT OF SHOCK

A. Classic signs of shock
   1. Altered level of consciousness (LOC) progressing to unresponsiveness
   2. Tachycardia progressing to absent pulses in decompensated/irreversible shock
   3. Pale, cool, clammy skin
   4. Normal BP during compensated shock and falling BP during decompensated shock

5. Differentiating compensated vs. decompensated shock
   i. Signs and symptoms of compensated shock
      - Tachycardia (usually the first sign in adults)
      - Altered LOC (restless, anxious, irritable)
      - Pale, cool, clammy skin
      - Thirst
      - **Normal** blood pressure
   ii. Signs and symptoms of decompensated shock
      - Decreased LOC
      - Absent peripheral pulses
      - Mottling, cyanosis
      - **Falling** blood pressure progressing to **hypotension**

> *Remember:* A tachycardic child with signs of shock may be close to cardiovascular collapse even if BP is normal. Hypotension is a **late** and **ominous** sign in pediatric patients.

B. Standard shock management
   1. Airway management, supplemental oxygen, ventilation support as indicated.
   2. Control bleeding as indicated.
   3. Consider tranexamic acid per local protocol. See Drug Profiles chapter.
   4. Prevent heat loss (even mild hypothermia increases metabolic demand and inhibits clotting).
   5. Rapid transport.
   6. IV access.
   7. Initiate early isotonic fluid resuscitation as indicated to maintain or restore adequate perfusion to vital organs.
      i. Rule out pulmonary edema before IV fluid bolus.
      ii. Fluid bolus not typically indicated for adults with SBP of at least 100 mmHg.

iii. If indicated (SBP 90 or below for adults), consider 250–500 mL fluid bolus as needed to achieve MAP of at least 60 mmHg.

iv. Burn patients: See Burn Injuries chapter.

v. Pediatric patients: See Pediatrics chapter.

8. Check lactate if possible (greater than 2 mmol/L is abnormal).

9. *Note:* There is no clear evidence that use of the pneumatic anti-shock garment is beneficial in managing shock.

C. Cardiogenic shock

1. Left ventricular failure due to myocardial infarction is the most common cause.

2. Signs and symptoms

   i. Classic signs of shock

   ii. Dyspnea and pulmonary edema

   iii. Cyanosis

3. Management

   i. Standard shock management.

   ii. Early, aggressive IV fluid administration is essential. If patient deteriorates after fluid administration (e.g., rales), withhold further fluid administration.

   iii. Vasopressors as needed to maintain/restore adequate perfusion to vital organs.

D. Hypovolemic shock

1. Causes include hemorrhage, vomiting, diarrhea, burns, sweating, diabetic ketoacidosis.

2. Signs and symptoms

   i. Classic signs of shock

3. Management

   i. Classic management

   ii. IV fluids

   ➤ IV fluids indicated for most causes of hypovolemic shock with presenting hypotension; however, specific guidelines vary and are still controversial (search "permissive hypotension" for additional info).

- ➤ Permissive hypotension
    - Research on permissive hypotension is currently inconclusive; however, there are indications of possible improved outcomes for patients whose BP is maintained at not greater than about 90 systolic.
    - Follow local protocols regarding IV fluid resuscitation for shock and trauma patients.
- ➤ Pediatric fluid resuscitation
    - Infants: 10 mL/kg
    - Children: 20 mL/kg

> ➤ **Remember:** Prehospital administration of tranexamic acid has shown benefit in patients treated within 1 hour of injury or with severe shock.
>
> — *JAMA Surgery* 2020 Li SR, Guyette F, Brown J, Zenati M, Reitz KM, Eastridge B, Nirula R, Vercruysse GA, O'Keeffe T, Joseph B, Neal MD, Zuckerbraun BS, Sperry JL. Early Prehospital Tranexamic Acid Following Injury Is Associated With a 30-day Survival Benefit: A Secondary Analysis of a Randomized Clinical Trial. Ann Surg. 2021 Sep 1;274(3):419–426. doi: 10.1097/SLA.0000000000005002. PMID: 34132695; PMCID: PMC8480233.

E. Neurogenic shock (a "warm" shock)
1. Damage to brain or spinal cord leading to widespread vasodilation and relative hypovolemia.
2. Signs and symptoms
    i. Possible paralysis (may be lower extremities or all extremities, and may include diaphragm).
    ii. Possible respiratory compromise (may indicate high cervical injury).
    iii. Mechanism of injury indicative of probable spinal injury.
    iv. Warm, flushed, dry skin (**not** the pale, cool, clammy skin usually seen).

Bleeding and Shock

      v. Hypotension even in early stage of shock.

      vi. Slow pulse (**not** the tachycardia usually seen).

      vii. *Note:* Three unique characteristics of neurogenic shock:

- Early hypotension.
- Bradycardia.
- Warm, dry skin.

    3. Management

      i. Standard shock management

F. Anaphylactic shock (a "warm" shock)

    1. Life-threatening allergic reaction to an antigen, such as food, meds, venom

    2. Signs and symptoms

      i. Skin: Flushed, itching, angioedema, urticaria

      ii. Respiratory: Dyspnea, wheezing, stridor, laryngospasm

      iii. Cardiovascular: Widespread vasodilation, tachycardia

    3. Management

      i. Aggressive airway intervention likely needed due to laryngospasm.

      ii. High-flow oxygen and ventilatory support as indicated.

      iii. Epinephrine.

      iv. IV fluids for volume support.

      v. Consider antihistamines and steroids per local protocol.

      vi. *Note:* Three acute life threats caused by anaphylaxis:

- Airway compromise (laryngospasm).
- Respiratory compromise (bronchoconstriction/edema).
- Circulatory compromise (massive vasodilation).

G. Septic shock/sepsis (a "warm" shock)

    1. Systemic infection that enters the blood and is carried throughout the body.

Chapter 6

    2. Primarily a "pipe" problem. Often leads to hypotension due to poor vasoconstriction, increased vessel permeability, fever, tachypnea, and poor fluid intake.

    3. Signs and symptoms

        i. Fever or hypothermia possible.

        ii. Skin can be flushed, pale, or cyanotic.

        iii. Altered LOC.

        iv. Dyspnea, abnormal lung sounds.

        v. Tachycardia, hypotension.

        vi. "Flash" capillary refill (less than 1 second) may be seen in early septic shock.

    4. Management

        i. Standard shock management and IV fluid support

H. Psychogenic shock

    1. A form of pseudo-shock causing acute, transient vasodilation that can cause syncopal episode.

    2. Does **not** cause sustained inadequate tissue perfusion.

    3. Always consider causes of syncope; maintain high index of suspicion for significant injuries or illnesses (shock, dehydration, dysrhythmia, hypoglycemia, hypoxia, etc.).

VII. MULTIPLE ORGAN DYSFUNCTION SYNDROME

A. Multiple organ failure following conditions such as shock, trauma, burns, surgery, renal failure.

B. Major cause of death following sepsis, significant trauma and major burns.

C. Early stages present with fever, altered LOC, tachycardia, dyspnea.

D. Later stages present with systems failure, moving from pulmonary to hepatic, intestinal, renal, and finally cardiac failure, encephalopathy, and death.

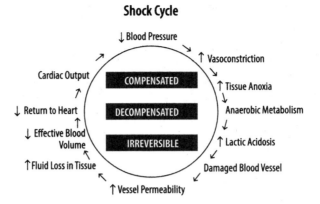

REVIEW QUESTIONS
(Answers on pg. 415.)

1. Which of the following are considered distributive shock? (Select THREE.)

   A. septic shock

   B. tension pneumothorax

   C. hemorrhagic shock

   D. anaphylactic shock

   E. neurogenic shock

   F. cardiac tamponade

2. Dark stool, a possible indication of internal bleeding, is known as:

   A. hematochezia.

   B. Grey Turner's sign.

   C. melena.

   D. urticaria.

Chapter 6

3. What is the single most preventable cause of traumatic death?

   A. external bleeding

   B. traumatic brain injury

   C. internal bleeding

   D. spinal injury

4. What are the three primary causes of shock? (Select THREE.)

   A. fluid loss

   B. increased intracranial pressure

   C. pump (heart) damage

   D. vasoconstriction

   E. hypoxia

   F. vasodilation

5. Which of the following is the best indication that your patient has entered decompensated shock?

   A. tachycardia

   B. restlessness

   C. coma

   D. falling blood pressure

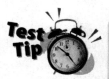

Security on the national certification exam is rigorous. The questions come from an extensive, unpublished database. There is no way to view these questions in advance. The keys to passing the exam are possession of the necessary knowledge and good test-taking skills. This book will help with both!

PART IV
MEDICAL EMERGENCIES
(Part 1)

Cardiology and Resuscitation

Chapter 7

CARDIOLOGY

I. TERMS TO KNOW

A. **Acute coronary syndrome:** Cardiac conditions caused by sudden, reduced blood flow to the heart. Includes myocardial infarction and unstable angina.

B. **Afterload:** Resistance the left heart overcomes during contraction.

C. **Aneurysm:** A weakening in the wall of an artery.

D. **Angina (stable):** Transient chest pain due to lack of oxygen to the myocardium. Typically exertional, and resolved by rest or nitroglycerin.

E. **Ascites:** Edema in the abdomen.

F. **Cardiac output:** Volume of blood ejected by left ventricle in 1 minute (stroke volume × heart rate).

G. **Compression fraction:** Percentage of time during patient resuscitation spent performing chest compressions. Cumulative time spent providing compressions divided by total time taken for entire resuscitation.

H. **Cor pulmonale:** Enlargement of the right side of the heart, often due to pulmonary hypertension.

I. **Diaphoresis:** Excessive sweating due to a secondary condition.

Chapter 7

J. **Inotrope:** Refers to effects on force of cardiac contraction. Positive inotropic agents increase force of cardiac contraction and negative inotropic agents decrease force of cardiac contraction.

K. **Myocardial infarction (MI):** Heart attack; aka acute myocardial infarction (AMI).

L. **Orthopnea:** Difficulty breathing while supine.

M. **Paroxysmal nocturnal dyspnea:** Acute onset of difficulty breathing at night, usually while sleeping.

N. **Silent MI:** Aka silent heart attack. An atypical AMI with no symptoms, minimal symptoms, or unrecognized symptoms.

O. **Stroke volume:** Amount of blood ejected by left ventricle during one contraction.

P. **Unstable angina:** Unpredictable angina that occurs without physical exertion, becomes more severe, and is unresponsive to nitroglycerin.

II. RISK FACTORS FOR HEART DISEASE

A. Smoking

B. Hypertension

C. Age (risk increases with age)

D. High cholesterol

E. Diabetes

F. Heredity

G. Sex (increased risk for males)

H. Substance abuse, especially cocaine

I. Lack of exercise

J. Oral contraceptives

K. Stress

III. ANATOMY & PHYSIOLOGY REVIEW

Note: See "Respiratory System" in the Anatomy & Physiology Review at *www.rea.com/paramedic*.

IV. ECG INTERPRETATION

A. Basic ECG interpretation cannot be adequately covered in this review text; however, here are the rhythm categories and dysrhythmias you should be familiar with:

1. Sinus rhythms and dysrhythmias
    i. Sinus rhythm
    ii. Sinus arrhythmia
    iii. Sinus bradycardia
    iv. Sinus tachycardia
    v. Sinus block
    vi. Sinus arrest
2. Atrial rhythms and dysrhythmias
    i. Supraventricular tachycardia
    ii. Paroxysmal supraventricular tachycardia
    iii. Atrial flutter
    iv. Atrial fibrillation
    v. Premature atrial complexes
    vi. Wandering atrial pacemaker
    vii. Multifocal atrial tachycardia

Chapter 7

    3. AV blocks
        i. First-degree AV block
        ii. Second-degree AV block type I
        iii. Second-degree AV block type II
        iv. Second-degree AV block 2:1 conduction
        v. Third-degree AV block
    4. Junctional rhythms and dysrhythmias
        i. Junctional escape rhythm
        ii. Junctional bradycardia
        iii. Accelerated junctional rhythm
        iv. Junctional tachycardia
        v. Premature junctional complexes
        vi. Junctional escape complexes
    5. Ventricular rhythms and dysrhythmias
        i. Accelerated idioventricular rhythm
        ii. Ventricular tachycardia
        iii. Ventricular fibrillation
        iv. Polymorphic ventricular tachycardia/Torsades de pointes
        v. Ventricular escape complexes
        vi. Ventricular escape rhythm, aka idioventricular rhythm
        vii. Ventricular escape complexes
        viii. Premature ventricular complexes
    6. Additional rhythms and dysrhythmias
        i. Asystole
        ii. Artificial pacemaker rhythms

B. 12-lead ECG: See Patient Monitoring Technology chapter for a review on 12-lead ECG.

Cardiology and Resuscitation

V. COMMON SIGNS AND SYMPTOMS OF CARDIAC EMERGENCIES

A. Chest pain or pressure

B. Dyspnea

C. Palpitations

D. Diaphoresis

E. Restlessness, anxiety

F. Feeling of impending doom

G. Nausea and vomiting

H. Generalized weakness or flu-like symptoms

I. Edema

J. Denial or feeling of impending doom

K. Pallor

VI. GENERAL MANAGEMENT OF CARDIAC EMERGENCIES

A. Assess and manage ABCs (Airway, Breathing, Circulation).

B. Basic life support (BLS) and advanced cardiac life support (ACLS) interventions as indicated for cardiac arrest.

C. Supplemental oxygen as indicated to maintain SpO_2 of at least 94%.

D. Continuous ECG monitoring and serial 12-lead ECG.

Chapter 7

    E. IV access and pharmacological interventions as indicated (Examples: aspirin, nitroglycerin).

    F. Rapid transport to the closest appropriate facility.

VII. MANAGEMENT OF CARDIAC DYSRHYTHMIAS

    A. Determine if patient is symptomatic, e.g., altered level of consciousness (LOC), hypotensive, chest pain, etc.

    B. Follow appropriate ACLS algorithm.

        1. Consider vagal maneuvers for tachydysrhythmias.

        2. Consider appropriate pharmacological interventions.

        3. Consider appropriate electrical interventions, e.g., cardioversion, defibrillation, transcutaneous external pacing.

VIII. ACUTE CORONARY SYNDROME (ACS)

        1. ACS includes *unstable* angina, ST-elevation MI (STEMI), and non-ST elevation MI (NSTEMI).

IX. ANGINA

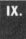

    A. Aka "stable" angina or "typical" angina.

    B. Transient chest pain due to myocardial ischemia.

    C. Often provoked by exertion or stress.

    D. Typically lasts less than 15 minutes and resolves with rest or nitroglycerin.

    E. Most common ECG finding is ST depression.

    F. *Note:* Considered a chronic condition, not ACS.

X. UNSTABLE ANGINA

A. Presents with at least *one* of the following:
1. New-onset angina.
2. Angina for at least 20 minutes while at rest.
3. Frequent angina episodes or increasing duration of angina.

XI. ACUTE MYOCARDIAL INFARCTION (AMI)

A. AMI is irreversible necrosis of myocardial muscle and diagnosed by ECG changes and elevated cardiac biomarkers.

B. AMI classification is based on ECG findings.
1. ST-elevation MI (STEMI)
2. Non-ST-elevation MI (NSTEMI)

C. "Silent" MI
1. An atypical AMI with no symptoms, minimal symptoms, or unrecognized symptoms.
2. About 30%–45% of myocardial infarctions may be silent MI.
3. Signs and symptoms may include:
    i. Indigestion.
    ii. Flu-like symptoms, fatigue.
    iii. Complaint of muscle strain-type pain in chest, upper back, or arm.
    iv. Neck or jaw pain.
4. High-risk populations for silent MI
    i. Women (***Note:*** Some data suggests silent MI may be more common in men, but more fatal in women.)
    ii. Diabetics
    iii. Elderly

Chapter 7

> ➤ **Remember:** Consider right ventricular infarct, pulmonary embolism, and cardiac tamponade for any patient with jugular vein distention (JVD), clear lungs, and hypotension.

D. Right ventricular infarctions
   1. About 40% of inferior wall infarctions involve the right ventricle.
   2. Use caution when considering nitroglycerin in suspected right ventricular MI (risk of profound hypotension). Follow local protocol.
   3. Consider an IV fluid bolus for suspected right ventricular infarction (without pulmonary edema) to help maintain hemodynamic stability (per local protocol).

XII. CONGESTIVE HEART FAILURE (CHF)

A. Left heart failure
   1. Left ventricular dysfunction causes backpressure into pulmonary circulation.
   2. Dyspnea and pulmonary edema are common with left heart failure.
   3. Myocardial infarction is a common cause of left heart failure.

B. Right heart failure
   1. Right ventricular dysfunction causes backpressure into systemic venous circulation.
   2. JVD and pedal edema are common with right heart failure.
   3. Left heart failure and cor pulmonale are common causes of right heart failure.

> ➤ **Remember:** Always assess cardiac and respiratory patients for JVD. Consider the following potential causes of abnormal JVD (especially if accompanied by hypotension): Clear lung sounds: Right heart failure, pulmonary embolism, cardiac tamponade. Absent lung sounds: Tension pneumothorax.

C. Signs and symptoms of CHF
1. Pulmonary edema (typically left heart failure)
2. Dyspnea (typically left heart failure)
3. Paroxysmal nocturnal dyspnea (typically left heart failure)
4. Orthopnea (typically left heart failure)
5. Mottled skin
6. Weakness
7. Ascites (typically right heart failure)
8. JVD (typically right heart failure)
9. Bilateral pedal edema (typically right heart failure)
10. *Note:* Patients with a history of CHF are often prescribed medications such as digoxin (positive inotrope), a diuretic (such as furosemide), an ACE inhibitor, and a potassium supplement.
11. *Note:* Be very clear on the signs and symptoms that distinguish left vs. right heart failure—and remember, some patients can have bilateral heart failure.

Left Heart Failure	Right Heart Failure
• Dyspnea	• JVD
• Pulmonary edema	• Pedal edema

Figure 7-2.

D. Management of CHF
1. Avoid placing patient supine.
2. Supplemental oxygen as indicated.
3. Continuous positive airway pressure (CPAP) as indicated starting with 5 cm H_2O and up to 10 cm H_2O if needed.
4. ECG monitoring.
5. IV access.
6. Nitroglycerin as indicated.
7. Use of narcotics and diuretics in the treatment of acute CHF patients has been shown to be ineffective and possibly harmful.

Chapter 7

XIII. CARDIAC TAMPONADE

A. Aka pericardial tamponade.

B. Excess fluid accumulation in the pericardial sac impairing diastolic filling and reducing cardiac output.

C. Causes can be medical or trauma related.

D. Signs and symptoms

1. Chest pain

2. Dyspnea and orthopnea

3. Beck's triad: JVD, narrowing pulse pressure (hypotension), muffled heart tones (*Note:* Muffled heart sounds occur late.)

4. *Note:* For any patient with JVD and clear lung sounds: Be alert for possible right ventricular infarct, pulmonary embolism, or cardiac tamponade.

E. Management

1. High-flow oxygen

2. IV fluids if hypotensive

3. Consider vasopressors, such as dopamine

4. Rapid transport

XIV. HYPERTENSIVE EMERGENCIES

A. Signs and symptoms

1. Elevation in blood pressure (>180/120) with some sort of target organ change, such as:

    i. Altered LOC

    ii. Headache

    iii. Dyspnea

    iv. Chest pain

    v. Vomiting

vi. Visual disturbance

vii. Pulmonary edema

viii. ECG changes

ix. Symptoms of stroke

x. Seizures

2. History of hypertensive disorder

3. Noncompliance with antihypertensive meds

4. Pregnancy (preeclampsia and pregnancy-induced hypertension, which may occur up to 3 weeks postpartum)

5. Nose bleed

B. Management

1. Manage airway, breathing, circulation as indicated.

2. Supplemental oxygen as indicated.

3. Place in position of comfort (pregnant patients left lateral recumbent).

4. IV access (do not delay transport to establish IV).

5. Transport.

XV. ABDOMINAL AORTIC ANEURYSM (AAA)

A. Aortic aneurysms often occur in the abdominal region, but can also develop along the thoracic aorta (thoracic aortic aneurysm) or in the brain (cerebral aneurysm).

B. The weakened wall of the affected artery is prone to rupture and massive bleeding.

C. Signs and symptoms of AAA

1. Most common in males between 40 and 60 years old.

2. Tearing abdominal, back, or flank pain.

3. Possible history of hypertension, smoking, atherosclerosis, family history of AAA.

4. Possible pulsating abdominal mass.

5. Varying blood pressures between left and right arms of at least 15 mmHg.
6. Signs and symptoms of hypovolemic shock (if ruptured).

D. Management
1. General management of advanced life support patients.
2. Keep patient still.
3. Caution when palpating abdomen.
4. Transport rapidly to appropriate facility with surgical capabilities.

XVI. CARDIOGENIC SHOCK

A. Persistent, severe left ventricular pump failure despite correction of existing dysrhythmias, hypovolemia, or widespread vasodilation.

B. Frequently caused by massive MI; can also be caused by tension pneumothorax, cardiac tamponade, or pulmonary embolism.

C. Signs and symptoms
1. Hypotension (may be <80 mmHg systolic)
2. Tachycardia
3. Chest pain
4. Dyspnea
5. Altered LOC
6. Weakness
7. History of trauma or MI

D. Management
1. Manage airway, breathing, circulation as indicated.
2. Position of comfort if possible.
3. Oxygen as indicated.
4. Consider CPAP.
5. Consider vasopressor medication, such as dopamine.
6. Rapid transport to appropriate facility.

Cardiology and Resuscitation

XVII. SPECIAL CONSIDERATIONS

A. Automatic implantable cardioverter-defibrillators (AICD)

1. An AICD is like an automated external defibrillator (AED) but is placed under the skin and connected directly to the heart.

2. The energy level from an AICD is much lower than from an external defibrillator, so it presents minimal risk of injury to rescuers.

3. Treat as you would any other patient; however, if applying multipurpose defib/pacer pads, do not place pads directly over device.

B. Pacemaker

1. An implanted device that helps regulate a patient's cardiac rate by serving as an artificial source of electrical impulses to stimulate the heart.

2. Patients with malfunctioning pacemaker often experience dizziness, weakness, bradycardia, and hypotension.

3. Assess ECG. Provide supportive care per local protocol.

4. If applying multipurpose defib/pacer pads, do not place pads directly over device.

C. Ventricular assist device (VAD)

1. Implanted mechanical device that replaces the function of the ventricles for patients with a failing heart. May be a temporary treatment or permanent.

2. Most VADs produce continuous flow, so the patient may not have a palpable pulse or measurable blood pressure.

3. Look for cable from abdominal wall connecting to the device.

4. SpO_2 may be inaccurate. Use mental status and skin condition to assess perfusion and oxygenation.

5. Patient and family will be knowledgeable about VAD and will have contact info for VAD coordinator. Consult the VAD coordinator for help.

6. Consult medical direction for appropriate destination.

7. Most common malfunction is low batteries or battery failure. Keep the batteries and controller with the patient.

8. If applying multipurpose defib/pacer pads, do not place pads directly over device.

9. You do not need to disconnect VAD to defibrillate or acquire 12-lead ECG.

10. Perform CPR if pump has stopped and patient is unresponsive with no signs of life.

11. Do not perform CPR if pump is still functioning (assess patient and auscultate for pump "hum"). Ventricular fibrillation (VF)/ventricular tachycardia (VT) or asystole may be patient's "normal" underlying rhythm.

12. Administer IV fluids for hypotension.

13. Many VAD patients also have an AICD.

> *Remember:* Research shows EMS agencies with higher rates of on-scene resuscitation for out-of-hospital cardiac arrest have higher return of spontaneous circulation (ROSC), increased overall survival rates, and favorable neurological outcomes.
>
> — *Resuscitation* 2021;169:205–213

RESUSCITATION

I. EXAM GUIDELINES

A. The national certification exam is based on the current American Heart Association (AHA) guidelines for Basic Life Support, Emergency Cardiovascular Care, and Advanced Cardiovascular Life Support.

II. HIGHLIGHTS OF CURRENT AHA BLS GUIDELINES

A. Rate of chest compression: 100–120 per minute (adults and peds).

B. Depth of compression: adults: 2"–2.4" (5–6 cm).

C. Depth of compression: children: 2" (5 cm) or 1/3 depth of the chest for all pediatric patients (infants and children).

Cardiology and Resuscitation

D. Depth of compression: infants: 1.5" (4 cm) 1/3 depth of the chest for all pediatric patients (infants and children).

E. Adult compression to ventilation ratio: 30:2 (one or two rescuer).

F. Infant and child compression to ventilation ratio: 30:2 (one rescuer), 15:2 (two rescuer).

G. Ventilation rate with advanced airway: 10/minute (adults), 20–30/minute (children).

H. Ensure full chest recoil between compressions.

I. Minimize interruptions in chest compressions (less than 10 seconds) to maintain compression fraction of greater than 80%.

J. Avoid hyperventilation.

K. Utilize AED to determine need for defibrillation as early as possible.

L. Oxygen should be administered to maintain SpO_2 of at least 94% (but less than 100% after ROSC).

M. Evidence does not demonstrate benefit of mechanical CPR devices over manual CPR.

N. Routine suctioning of newborns not indicated.

III. HIGHLIGHTS OF CURRENT AHA ACLS GUIDELINES

A. Vasopressin not recommended for cardiac arrest.

B. Amiodarone or lidocaine may be used for efractory VF or pulseless VT after three defib attempts and epinephrine.

C. Consider termination of efforts if unable to obtain $ETCO_2$ above 10 mmHg in an intubated patient after 20 minutes of CPR.

D. Atropine indicated for symptomatic bradycardia (altered LOC, chest pain, hypotension).

Chapter 7

    E. Consider dopamine or epinephrine infusion or transcutaneous external pacing (TEP) for symptomatic bradycardia unresponsive to atropine.

    F. Consider immediate TEP for symptomatic bradycardia with high-degree AV block when IV access delayed.

    G. 12-lead ECG should be obtained prehospital for suspected acute coronary syndrome to assess for STEMI.

IV. HIGHLIGHTS OF CURRENT AHA PEDIATRIC ADVANCED LIFE SUPPORT (PALS) GUIDELINES

    A. Early, rapid administration of isotonic IV fluids at 20 mL/kg recommended for pediatric patients with hypovolemia or sepsis.

    B. Amiodarone or lidocaine can be used for shock-refractory VF or pulseless VT.

    C. Administer oxygen as indicated to maintain SpO_2 between 94% and 99%.

    D. Cuffed endotracheal tubes are recommended for pediatric patients.

V. SPECIAL SITUATIONS

    A. Pregnant patients

       1. Prone to hypoxia, so aggressive airway management and oxygenation is indicated.

       2. Provide continuous lateral uterine displacement for pregnant patients in cardiac arrest.

    B. Hypothermic patients in cardiac arrest

       1. May be unresponsive to defibrillation. Only one defibrillation attempt is recommended for VF/VT. Follow local protocol.

       2. Only one dose of drug therapy is recommended. Medications can accumulate to toxic levels in peripheral circulation. Follow local protocol.

3. Intubation and ventilation with warm, humidified oxygen is recommended.

4. Provide basic maneuvers to limit heat loss.

5. Only withhold resuscitation if the patient has obvious lethal injuries or if the body is frozen so that nose and mouth are blocked by ice and chest compressions are not possible.

C. Mechanical CPR devices

1. CPR devices (Lucas, AutoPulse, etc.) provide consistent rate and depth of compression.

2. Can free up rescuers for other tasks.

3. No current evidence that mechanical CPR devices improve survival rates compared to manual CPR.

4. Follow local protocol regarding use of mechanical CPR devices.

REVIEW QUESTIONS
(Answers on pg. 415.)

1. The resistance the heart overcomes during contraction is known as:

    A. afterload.

    B. preload.

    C. cardiac output.

    D. minute volume.

2. Which of the following is the heart's primary pacemaker?

    A. ventricles

    B. bundle of His

    C. sinoatrial node

    D. atrioventricular node

Chapter 7

3. Acute coronary syndrome includes which of the following? (Select THREE.)
   A. all chest pain
   B. unstable angina
   C. stable angina
   D. STEMI
   E. NSTEMI
   F. cardiogenic shock

4. Which of the following are most likely if your patient presents with JVD, clear lung sounds, and hypotension? (Select THREE.)
   A. left heart failure
   B. tension pneumothorax
   C. pulmonary embolism
   D. cardiac tamponade
   E. hypovolemic shock
   F. right ventricular infarct

5. Which of the following assessments will help the paramedic distinguish left heart failure from right heart failure? (Select THREE.)
   A. lung sounds
   B. JVD
   C. standard ECG
   D. pedal edema
   E. heart tones
   F. ascites

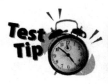

Search online for the American Heart Association document titled "Highlights of the American Heart Association Guidelines for CPR and ECC." This is a gold mine of study material related to BLS, ACLS, and PALS content you can expect to see on the certification exam.

Pulmonology

I. TERMS TO KNOW

A. **Acute respiratory distress syndrome (ARDS):** Noncardiogenic pulmonary edema.

B. **Forced expiratory volume (FEV):** Volume of air that can be exhaled from a full inhalation by exhaling forcefully and rapidly for a timed period.

C. **Hemoptysis:** Coughing up blood.

D. **Minute volume:** Respiratory rate × tidal volume.

E. **Peak expiratory flow (PEF):** Measurement of air flowing in and out of the lungs.

F. **Positive end-expiratory pressure (PEEP):** Extrinsic PEEP uses an impedance valve to increase volume of air remaining in lungs at end of expiration to improve gas exchange.

G. **Subcutaneous emphysema:** Crackling under the skin upon palpation due to trapped air. Typically found in chest, neck, or face.

H. **Tidal volume:** Volume of air inhaled or exhaled with each breath.

II. ANATOMY & PHYSIOLOGY REVIEW

Note: See "Respiratory System" in the online Anatomy & Physiology Review at *www.rea.com/paramedic*.

Chapter 8

 III. GENERAL SIGNS AND SYMPTOMS OF RESPIRATORY COMPROMISE

    A. Positional breathing, such as tripod breathing

    B. Skin color changes, such as cyanosis

    C. Altered level of consciousness (LOC)

    D. Difficulty speaking full sentences

    E. Difficulty breathing

    F. Accessory muscle use, e.g., nasal flaring, intercostal retractions, tracheal tugging

    G. Abnormal respiratory rate or tidal volume

    H. SpO_2 below 94%

    I. Abnormal lung sounds

 IV. GENERAL MANAGEMENT OF RESPIRATORY COMPROMISE

    A. Manage ABCs (Airway, Breathing, Circulation) as indicated.

    B. Monitor SpO_2.

    C. Monitor $ETCO_2$ as indicated.

    D. Monitor ECG.

    E. Provide supplemental oxygen if hypoxia suspected and as indicated to maintain SpO_2 of 94%–99%.

    F. IV access, as indicated.

    G. Support ventilations as indicated ($ETCO_2$ of 35–45 mmHg).

H. Consider causes, e.g., various respiratory or cardiac problems, trauma, sepsis, etc.

I. Consider continuous positive airway pressure (CPAP) as indicated.

J. Consider pharmacologic interventions as indicated.

K. Transport.

V. SPECIFIC RESPIRATORY EMERGENCIES

A. Foreign body airway obstruction

1. Follow current American Heart Association Basic Life Support guidelines for complete or severe airway obstruction.

    i. Conscious adults and children: Continuous abdominal thrusts until the obstruction is relieved or the patient becomes unconscious.

    ii. Conscious infant: Alternating back slaps and chest thrusts until the obstruction is relieved or the patient becomes unconscious.

    iii. Unconscious patient: Begin CPR.

B. Acute respiratory distress syndrome (ARDS)

1. ARDS is a form of pulmonary edema **not** caused by poor left ventricular function. There are many causes, including sepsis, trauma, overdose, drowning, toxic inhalation.

2. Signs and symptoms

    i. Progressive decline in respiratory status

    > *Note:* Acute-onset respiratory failure in healthy patient may indicate high-altitude pulmonary edema (HAPE).

    ii. Dyspnea

    iii. Altered LOC, such as agitation, confusion

    iv. Fatigue

    v. Pulmonary edema (rales bilaterally)

    vi. Tachypnea

vii. Tachycardia

viii. Possible cyanosis

ix. Low SpO_2

3. Management

   i. See General Management of Respiratory Compromise with emphasis on:
      - Monitor SpO_2.
      - Position patient upright, legs dangling.
      - Rapid descent to lower altitude if HAPE suspected.
      - Consider CPAP, with PEEP.

C. Chronic obstructive pulmonary disease (COPD)

   1. Pathophysiology

      i. Slowly progressive respiratory disease with high mortality rates

      ii. Includes emphysema and chronic bronchitis

      iii. Typically caused by smoking and environmental toxins

   2. Signs and symptoms

      i. Possible history of smoking or exposure to cigarette smoke

      ii. Cough with increased mucus production

      iii. Air trapping with prolonged expiratory phase

      iv. Signs of right heart failure, including jugular vein distention and pedal edema

      v. Chronic dyspnea, worsening on exertion

      vi. Tachypnea

      vii. Accessory muscle use

      viii. Possible flushed or cyanotic skin

      ix. Pursed-lip breathing

      x. Low SpO_2

      xi. Abnormal lung sounds, such as diminished, rhonchi

      xii. Clubbing of the fingers

3. Management
   i. See General Management of Respiratory Compromise.
   ii. Special considerations:
      ➤ COPD patients may have chronically low SpO_2; target oxygen administration to an SpO_2 of about 94%.
      ➤ Only a small percentage of COPD patients are on a hypoxic drive. Do **not** withhold oxygen from a COPD patient with signs of hypoxia, and monitor respiratory effort, rate, and tidal volume carefully.
      ➤ Bronchodilators such as albuterol or ipratropium are likely indicated.
      ➤ CPAP may help avoid progression to respiratory failure and need for intubation or bag-valve-mask ventilation.

D. Asthma
   1. Pathophysiology
      i. Chronic inflammatory airway disease.
      ii. Death rates rising, not falling.
      iii. About half of all asthma deaths occur before reaching the hospital.
      iv. Triggers include allergens, exercise, foods, stress, medications.
      v. An acute asthma attack will likely cause a decrease in peak flow and forced expiratory volume.
   2. Signs and symptoms
      i. Dyspnea
      ii. Wheezing
      iii. Cough
      iv. Pulsus paradoxus (drop in systolic BP of more than 10 mmHg during inspiration)
      v. Tachypnea
      vi. Tachycardia
      vii. Low SpO_2

3. Management
    i. See General Management of Respiratory Compromise.
    ii. Special considerations:
        ➤ Monitor peak expiratory flow (PEF) rates if possible.
        ➤ Aggressive use of bronchodilator medications (such as albuterol and ipratropium) are indicated to reverse bronchospasm.
4. Status asthmaticus
    i. Severe, prolonged asthma attack not reversible with bronchodilator medications.
    ii. Bronchoconstriction can be severe enough to cause absent lung sounds.
    iii. Respiratory arrest is often imminent, so aggressive treatment and rapid transport is indicated.

E. Pneumonia
  1. A lung infection, often leading to death in elderly and immunosuppressed patients
  2. Risk factors
      i. Chronic lung disease
      ii. Cerebral palsy
      iii. Living in a care facility
      iv. Dementia, stroke, neurological conditions
      v. Recent surgery
  3. Signs and symptoms
      i. Suspect pneumonia in any patient with a history of chest pain with associated fever, chills, or cough.
      ii. Weakness.
      iii. Cough.
      iv. Pleuritic chest pain.
      v. Dyspnea.
      vi. Tachypnea.
      vii. Abnormal lung sounds.

4. Management
    i. See General Management of Respiratory Compromise.
    ii. Dehydration is common; consider need for IV fluids.

F. Pulmonary embolism
   1. Pathophysiology
      i. Blockage (such as air, blood clot, amniotic fluid) in a pulmonary artery that decreases blood flow, leading to potentially fatal hypoxemia.
      ii. Risk factors
         ➤ Prolonged immobility of the extremities (such as a long flight)
         ➤ Recent surgery, especially major orthopedic surgery
         ➤ Long bone fracture
         ➤ Smoking
         ➤ Use of birth control medications
   2. Signs and symptoms
      i. Acute, unexplained dyspnea
      ii. Pleuritic chest pain
      iii. Cough, hemoptysis
      iv. Presence of risk factors listed above
      v. Tachypnea, often with normal lung sounds
      vi. Tachycardia
      vii. Possible indications of deep vein thrombosis (warm, swollen lower extremity with pain upon palpation or while extending calf)
      viii. Sudden cardiac arrest
   3. Management
      i. Aggressive oxygen therapy
      ii. Prepare for possible sudden cardiac arrest
      iii. Rapid transport

Chapter 8

- G. Spontaneous pneumothorax
    1. Pathophysiology
        i. Pneumothorax not related to blunt or penetrating trauma.
        ii. Recurrence rate is high (50%).
        iii. Much more common in males and smokers.
    2. Signs and symptoms
        i. Acute onset of sharp pleuritic chest pain or shoulder pain.
        ii. Possible localized diminished lung sounds.
        iii. Coughing fit or heavy lifting may precipitate symptoms.
        iv. Tachypnea
        v. Possible subcutaneous emphysema
    3. Management
        i. Closely monitor SpO_2.
        ii. Supplemental oxygen as indicated.
        iii. Transport in position of comfort.
- H. Hyperventilation syndrome
    1. Hyperventilation should be considered significant until confirmed otherwise. Anxiety is the most common cause, but there are many other dangerous possibilities.
    2. Signs and symptoms
        i. Tachypnea
        ii. Possible chest pain
        iii. Possible anxiety
        iv. Possible numbness
        v. Possible carpopedal spasm due to alkalosis and hypocalcemia
    3. Causes
        i. Anxiety (most common)
        ii. Metabolic disorders

iii. Respiratory disorders

iv. Pulmonary embolism

v. Cardiac disorders

vi. CNS disorders

vii. Various medications, e.g., aspirin

4. Management

    i. Supportive care.

    ii. Monitor SpO_2 and administer oxygen as indicated.

    iii. Transport.

    iv. **No** breathing into a paper bag, breath holding, or other attempts to raise the patient's CO_2 levels are recommended.

EMBOLISM

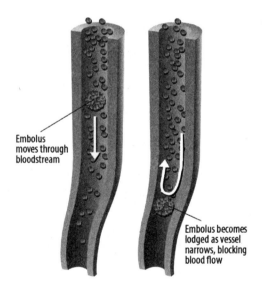

Figure 8-1.

Chapter 8

REVIEW QUESTIONS
(Answers on pg. 416.)

1. Your patient is coughing up blood. This is known as:
    A. hematemesis.
    B. ARDS.
    C. epistaxis.
    D. hemoptysis.

2. The exchange of gases (O_2, CO_2) between the circulatory system and the tissues of the body is known as:
    A. internal respiration.
    B. external respiration.
    C. spontaneous breathing.
    D. positive pressure ventilation.

3. Normal adult tidal volume (Vt) is about:
    A. 250 mL.
    B. 500 mL.
    C. 750 mL.
    D. 1,000 mL.

4. Oxygen should be administered as needed to maintain an SpO_2 of:
    A. 97%–100%.
    B. 94%–99%.
    C. 90%–94%.
    D. 88%–92%.

5. Your patient presents with sharp, pleuritic chest pain after attempting to lift a heavy object alone. You should suspect:

   A. aortic aneurysm.

   B. tension pneumothorax.

   C. spontaneous pneumothorax.

   D. pulmonary embolism.

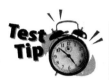

Use the information in this book to create flashcards for items that meet the following two criteria:

1. Important information you expect to see on the exam.

2. Information you need to study more before the exam.

Neurology

I. TERMS TO KNOW

A. **Ataxia:** Difficulty with coordinated movement.

B. **Decerebrate posturing:** Arms and legs extended.

C. **Decorticate posturing:** Arms flexed, legs extended.

D. **Dysphagia:** Difficulty swallowing.

E. **Hemiparesis:** Unilateral (one-sided) weakness.

F. **Hemiplegia:** Unilateral paralysis.

G. **Nuchal rigidity:** Inability of a patient to flex the head forward due to rigidity of the neck muscles. Often associated with meningitis.

H. **Nystagmus:** Involuntary eye movement.

II. ANATOMY & PHYSIOLOGY REVIEW

Note: See "Nervous System" in the online Anatomy & Physiology Review at *www.rea.com/paramedic*.

III. GENERAL SIGNS AND SYMPTOMS OF NERVOUS SYSTEM EMERGENCIES

A. Altered mentation, e.g. less than a score of 15 on the Glasgow Coma Scale (GCS). *Note:* this is frequently the hallmark characteristic of a neurological medical emergency.

Chapter 9

    B. Abnormal vitals, such as irregular respirations

    C. Cognitive, speech, motor, or sensory deficits (such as weakness, paralysis, slurred speech, confusion, etc.)

    D. Posturing (decorticate, decerebrate)

    E. Signs of increased intracranial pressure (ICP)
        1. Cushing's reflex: Systolic hypertension, bradycardia, irregular breathing
        2. Posturing: Decorticate or decerebrate

IV. GENERAL MANAGEMENT OF NEUROLOGIC EMERGENCIES

    A. Manage ABCs (Airway, Breathing, Circulation) as indicated.

    B. Monitor SpO_2 (94%–99%) and $ETCO_2$ (target 35–45 mmHg).

    C. Do **not** hyperventilate over 20 breaths/minute.

    D. Aggressively correct and avoid even transient episodes of hypoxia or hypotension.

    E. Monitor ECG.

    F. Assess blood glucose and manage as indicated.

    G. Provide supplemental oxygen as indicated to maintain SpO_2 of at least 94%.

    H. Support ventilations as needed to maintain $ETCO_2$ of 35–45 mmHg.

    I. IV access, as indicated.

    J. Consider causes (AEIOU-TIPS).

    K. Rapid transport to appropriate facility as indicated.

V. SPECIFIC NEUROLOGIC EMERGENCIES

A. Altered mental status
   1. Common causes (AEIOU-TIPS)
      i. **A**cidosis, alcohol
      ii. **E**pilepsy
      iii. **I**nfection
      iv. **O**verdose
      v. **U**remia (blood infection, often kidney related)
      vi. **T**rauma, toxins, tumor
      vii. **I**nsulin
      viii. **P**sychological, poison
      ix. **S**troke, seizures, shock
   2. Use possible causes and patient history as clues to what assessment and interventions are needed (SpO_2, blood glucose, possible trauma, seizure history, etc.).
   3. Certain interventions should be at least considered for all patients with altered mentation.
      i. Are spinal precautions indicated?
      ii. Is supplemental oxygen indicated?
      iii. Is dextrose or thiamine indicated?
      iv. Is naloxone indicated?
      v. Is rapid transport to a specialty facility indicated?

B. Stroke
   1. Causes: ischemia (occlusion, embolus, thrombus) and hemorrhage
   2. Signs and symptoms of stroke
      i. Altered mentation (confusion, coma)
      ii. Slurred speech
      iii. Dysphagia
      iv. Facial droop

Mental Status Assessment—Adults

Glasgow Coma Scale (GSC)*

	1	2	3	4	5	6
Eyes	Does not open eyes	Opens eyes in response to painful stimuli	Opens eyes in response to voice	Opens eyes spontaneously	N/A	N/A
Verbal	Makes no sounds	Incomprehensible sounds	Utters inappropriate words	Confused, disoriented	Oriented, converses normally	N/A
Motor	Makes no movement	Extension to painful stimuli	Abnormal flexion to painful stimuli	Flexion/withdrawal to painful stimuli	Localizes painful stimuli	Obeys command

*GCS comprises three tests: eye, verbal, and motor responses. The lowest possible GCS score (sum) is 3 (deep coma or death), while the highest score is 15 (fully awake person).

Reference: Teasdlae G., Jennett B. Assessment of coma and impaired consciousness. A practical scale. Lancet 1974, 2: 81–84.

      v. Unilateral weakness or paralysis

      vi. Ataxia

      vii. Severe headache (more common with hemorrhagic stroke)

   3. Stroke scales/scoring systems

      i. Los Angeles Prehospital Stroke Screen

         ➤ Assesses blood glucose, facial droop, grip strength, arm drift.

      ii. Cincinnati Prehospital Stroke Scale

         ➤ Assesses speech, facial droop, arm drift.

         ➤ Any abnormality in above assessments indicates likelihood of stroke.

   4. Management of suspected stroke

      i. See General Management of Neurologic Emergencies.

      ii. Perform stroke assessment per local protocol.

      iii. Protect paralyzed patient from further harm.

      iv. Rapid transport to stroke center (per local protocol).

Neurology

C. Transient ischemic attack (TIA)
   1. Caused by temporary impaired blood flow to brain.
   2. Mimics stroke, but resolve within 24 hours with no permanent damage.
   3. May indicate elevated risk of impending stroke.
   4. Treat as possible stroke.

D. Seizures
   1. Types of seizures
      i. Generalized seizures
         ➤ Tonic-clonic (grand mal) seizures
            — General motor seizures with loss of consciousness.
            — Patient experiences respiratory paralysis during seizure activity.
            — Watch for excessive oral secretions, incontinence, nystagmus.
            — Phases of tonic-clonic seizures:
               • Aura: Sensation that a seizure may occur. Occurs prior to a loss of consciousness. Not every seizure has an aura phase.
               • Tonic: Muscle tension.
               • Clonic: Muscle spasm.
               • Postictal: Recovery phase. Patient progresses from unconsciousness to confusion to alertness.
         ➤ Status epilepticus
            — Prolonged tonic-clonic seizure (greater than 5 minutes) or two or more tonic-clonic seizures without the patient regaining consciousness in between.
            — Typically caused by problems with prescribed seizure medications, such as failure to take as prescribed.
            — Extremely dangerous due to prolonged apnea, acidosis, possible hypertension, and increased ICP.
            — Critical interventions include airway protection, oxygenation, positive pressure ventilation, and anticonvulsant medications per local protocol.

Chapter 9

- Absence (petit mal) seizures
  - Generalized seizure with brief loss of consciousness or awareness.
  - Absence seizures are idiopathic (unknown cause) and rarely occur in adult patients.
  - Respiratory paralysis does not occur during an absence seizure.
- Pseudoseizures
  - Psychological seizure.
  - No respiratory paralysis and no postictal phase.

  ii. Partial seizures
  - Simple partial (focal motor) seizures
    - Occurs only in one area of the body.
    - No loss of consciousness, but can progress to tonic-clonic seizure.
  - Complex partial (temporal lobe or psychomotor) seizures
    - Patients can experience a distinctive aura, such as déjà vu, strange taste or smell, or visual changes.
    - A focal impaired awareness seizure.
    - Patient will likely be unaware of surroundings and can have nonpurposeful movement or acute personality changes.
    - Does **not** involve convulsions, but **does** impair consciousness.

2. Assessment and management
   i. Question bystanders, when possible, to determine onset, possibility of trauma, history of seizures, drug or alcohol use, and diabetes, and to determine if patient likely experienced a seizure or a syncopal episode.
   ii. Protect airway (no tongue blades, bite blocks, etc.). Insertion of advanced airway not usually necessary.
   iii. Do not restrain patient during seizure, but protect from harm.
   iv. Oxygen and ventilatory support as indicated.
   v. Spinal precautions as indicated.

vi. Assess blood glucose.

vii. Anticonvulsant medications per local protocol.

3. Special considerations for pediatric patients

   i. Midazolam (intramuscular or intranasal) 0.2 mg/kg is the recommended medication and dose for pediatric seizures. Rectal administration of medications is not recommended.

   ii. Pediatric patients are often underdosed with midazolam and still seizing upon arrival at the hospital.

   iii. Research indicates in often takes EMS up to 14 minutes to administer the first dose of benzodiazepines to seizing pediatric patients. This is often due to attempts to establish intravenous (IV)/intraosseous (IO) access or dose uncertainty.

   iv. IV access is not required for initial management of seizures. Do not delay administration of IM/IN benzodiazepines to establish IV/IO access.

> ***Remember:*** Consider meningitis or encephalitis for pediatric patients under 6 months or over 6 years who present with seizures and fever. This presentation is not consistent with febrile seizures.

E. Syncope

1. Fainting caused by temporary lack of blood flow to the brain

2. Consider common causes

   i. Cardiovascular conditions

   ii. Hypovolemia

   iii. Orthostatic hypotension

   iv. Diabetic problem

   v. TIA

   vi. Head injury

3. Management

   i. Spinal precautions as indicated.

   ii. Supplemental oxygen as indicated.

   iii. Assess vitals, ECG, blood glucose.

Chapter 9

      iv. IV access as indicated.

      v. Transport as indicated.

F. Headache

1. Common causes

    i. Vascular headaches, such as migraines and cluster headaches

    - Migraine headache
        - Severe throbbing pain on one or both sides of the head.
        - Can be preceded by an aura.
        - Often accompanied by nausea & vomiting; eye pain; hypersensitivity to light, sound, smell, touch.
    - Cluster headache
        - Severe headaches, usually on one side of the head, that occur in clusters.
        - Usually localized around the eye and accompanied by watering of the eye and nasal congestion.

    ii. Tension headaches

    - The most common cause of headaches, often triggered by stress.
    - Mild to severe pain to head, neck, or eyes.

    iii. Organic headaches, such as infections and tumors

    - Not a common cause of headaches.
    - Can be caused by cerebral neoplasm (brain tumor) or meningitis.
    - *Note:* Meningitis patients often present with throbbing headache, fever, and nuchal rigidity (neck stiffness).

2. Indications of possible serious condition include:

    i. Headache with associated fever and nuchal rigidity.

    ii. Headache in patient over 50 or under 5 years of age.

    iii. Complaint of "worst headache ever experienced."

iv. Headache with signs and symptoms of stroke.

v. Headache associated with exertion, coughing, sneezing, sex.

3. Management

i. Supplemental oxygen if indicated.

ii. IV access as indicated.

iii. Assess blood glucose.

iv. Monitor ECG, vitals.

v. Be prepared for possible vomiting, loss of consciousness.

vi. Transport as indicated.

G. Cranial nerve–related conditions

1. Bell's palsy: Sudden, unilateral weakness or paralysis of facial muscles.

2. Trigeminal neuralgia: Painful spasms, usually to one side of the face.

H. Degenerative neurological disorders

1. Alzheimer's disease: The most common cause of dementia.

2. Muscular dystrophy: Progressive muscle weakness and degeneration of skeletal muscle.

3. Multiple sclerosis: CNS and autoimmune disease. Causes weakness, sensory loss, paresthesia, vision changes.

4. Guillain-Barre syndrome: Immune system mistakenly attacks peripheral nerves, causing muscle weakness. Can cause ascending paralysis starting in the legs, leading to need for ventilatory support.

5. Parkinson's disease: Chronic and progressive disorder causing tremors, rigidity, bradykinesia (slow, impaired movement), poor balance and coordination.

6. Spina bifida: Fetal vertebrae do not close properly during pregnancy, leaving part of spine exposed. Nerve damage is permanent, and associated learning disabilities are common.

REVIEW QUESTIONS
(Answers on pg. 417.)

1. During your assessment, you determine that your patient is unable to flex her head forward (chin to chest). This is known as:
   A. hyperextension.
   B. hemiplegia.
   C. dysphagia.
   D. nuchal rigidity.

2. This is the largest part of the brain and controls thought, learning, memory, and senses:
   A. cerebrum.
   B. cerebellum.
   C. diencephalon.
   D. brainstem.

3. What is the outermost layer of the meninges?
   A. dura mater
   B. arachnoid layer
   C. pia mater
   D. pos

4. The "A" in AEIOU-TIPS stands for (select TWO):
   A. antidysrhythmics.
   B. acidosis.
   C. alcohol.
   D. allergies.
   E. antipyretic.

5. Your patient only opens his eyes in response to painful stimulus. His speech is incomprehensible, and he has abnormal extension. What is this patient's GCS?

   A. 3

   B. 6

   C. 12

   D. 15

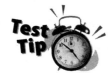

The questions on the national certification exam (and in this book and the accompanying digital practice exam) are based on the current National EMS Education Standards, not state or local protocols. This book should serve as an excellent resource, but it should not be your **only** resource.

Chapter 10

Endocrinology

I. TERMS TO KNOW

A. **HHNC:** Hyperglycemic hyperosmolar nonketotic coma.

B. **HHS:** Hyperosmolar hyperglycemic state.

C. **Kussmaul respirations:** Deep, rapid respirations.

D. **Polydipsia:** Excessive thirst.

E. **Polyphagia:** Excessive hunger.

F. **Polyuria:** Excessive urination.

II. ANATOMY & PHYSIOLOGY REVIEW

Note: See "Endocrine System" in the online Anatomy & Physiology Review at *www.rea.com/paramedic.*

III. DIABETES

A. Caused by inadequate insulin, which is required for normal blood glucose levels.

B. Type 1 diabetes
1. Little to no insulin production by the pancreas.
2. Aka juvenile diabetes or insulin-dependent diabetes.

3. Less common than type 2 diabetes but higher risk of complications, fatality.
4. Typically, type 1 diabetics require regular insulin injections.

C. Type 2 diabetes
1. Aka non-insulin-dependent diabetes. (*Note:* Some type 2 diabetics may require insulin.)
2. Obesity (and likely heredity) increase risk of type 2 diabetes.
3. Far more common than type 1 diabetes, but potentially manageable with diet, exercise, or oral hypoglycemic meds.

D. Diabetic ketoacidosis (DKA)
1. DKA is a life-threatening hyperglycemic complication of type 1 diabetes characterized by extremely high blood glucose levels (typically 400 mg/dL or higher).
2. Causes
   i. May be initial presentation of undiagnosed type 1 diabetes.
   ii. Failure to take insulin as indicated.
   iii. Physiologic stress, such as infection, surgery.
3. Signs and symptoms
   i. Elevated blood glucose levels
   ii. Polydipsia, polyphagia, polyuria
   iii. Decreased level of consciousness (LOC)
   iv. Warm, dry skin
   v. Nausea & vomiting, abdominal pain
   vi. Kussmaul respirations
   vii. Fruity or acetone odor on breath
   viii. Incontinence
   ix. *Note:* DKA has a **slow** onset of symptoms.
4. Management
   i. General management of advanced life support (ALS) patients (Patient Assessment chapter).

ii. Intravenous (IV) fluids for dehydration, hypovolemia.

iii. Insulin indicated, but typically **not** administered prehospital.

iv. Rapid transport.

E. Insulin shock

1. A life-threatening hypoglycemic emergency characterized by low blood glucose level (typically below 60 mg/dL).

2. *Note:* Insulin shock has a **rapid** onset, since the brain does not tolerate a lack of glucose for any length of time.

3. Signs and symptoms

   i. Low blood glucose levels

   ii. Altered LOC (restless, irritable, combative, coma)

   iii. Seizures

   iv. Cool, clammy skin

4. Management

   i. General management of ALS patients (Patient Assessment chapter).

   ii. Dextrose IV or glucagon intramuscular.

   ➤ Dextrose 10% can be administered safely to patients of all ages and works as effectively as other concentrations.

   ➤ Dextrose 25% can be used for patients that are at least 1 month of age; however, it is not preferred over dextrose 10%.

   ➤ Dextrose 50% can cause severe tissue necrosis upon extravasation and should not be carried by EMS.

   ➤ See dose table (Table 10-1).

   iii. Transport.

F. Hyperosmolar hyperglycemic state (HHS)

1. Also known as hyperglycemic hyperosmolar nonketotic coma (HHNC).

2. Potentially life-threatening complication of type 2 diabetes.

3. Characterized by prolonged hyperglycemia and severe dehydration.

Chapter 10

Table 10-1: Dextrose Dose Table

Dose (mg/kg)	Dextrose %	Volume (mL/kg)
0.5 gram/kg	Dextrose 25%	2 mL/kg
	Dextrose 10%	5 mL/kg
1 gram/kg	Dextrose 25%	4 mL/kg
	Dextrose 10%	10 mL/kg

4. Signs and symptoms
    i. Severe hyperglycemia (up to 1,000 mg/dL).
    ii. Diabetic history.
    iii. Altered LOC.
    iv. Signs and symptoms of dehydration.
    v. Increased urinary output.
    vi. *Note:* HHS (like DKA) has a **slow** onset; however, the patient does not have fruity or acetone breath.
5. Management
    i. Same as DKA (difficult to distinguish in prehospital setting).

G. Glucometry: See Electronic Patient Monitoring Technology chapter.

IV. MISCELLANEOUS ENDOCRINE DISORDERS

A. Pancreatitis
  1. Inflammation of the pancreas, typically due to gallstones or chronic alcohol abuse.
  2. Signs and symptoms
      i. Dull, constant flank pain. Typically worsens if supine.
      ii. Fever.
      iii. Jaundice.
      iv. Nausea & vomiting.

3. Management
    i. General management of ALS patients (Patient Assessment chapter).
    ii. Pain management.
    iii. Transport.

B. Graves' disease
   1. Excessive production of thyroid hormones.
   2. Signs and symptoms
       i. Emotional changes
       ii. Insomnia
       iii. Weight loss
       iv. Sensitivity to heat
       v. Weakness
       vi. Dyspnea
       vii. Tachycardia
       viii. New-onset atrial fibrillation (a-fib)
       ix. Protruding eyes
       x. Goiter
   3. Management
       i. General management of ALS patients (Patient Assessment chapter).
       ii. Consider beta-blockers as indicated for a-fib (per local protocol).
       iii. Consider dexamethasone (per local protocol).

C. Thyroid storm
   1. Life-threatening emergency, characterized by severe hypermetabolic state.
   2. Signs and symptoms
       i. Increased stimulation of sympathetic nervous system (fight or flight)
       ii. High fever

- iii. Altered LOC
- iv. Tachycardia
- v. Hypertension
- vi. Vomiting, diarrhea
3. Management
    - i. General management of ALS patients (Patient Assessment chapter).
    - ii. Rapid transport.

D. Myxedema
  1. Hypothyroidism characterized by low metabolic state and thickening of connective tissue.
  2. Signs and symptoms
      - i. Fatigue, lethargy
      - ii. Cold intolerance
      - iii. Slowed mental function or lack of emotion
      - iv. Puffy face
      - v. Decreased appetite and weight gain
      - vi. Coma
      - vii. Respiratory depression
  3. Management
      - i. General management of ALS patients (Patient Assessment chapter).
      - ii. Limit IV fluids.
      - iii. Avoid active rewarming.
      - iv. Transport.

E. Cushing's syndrome
  1. Adrenal disorder caused by hyperadrenalism (high cortisol levels).
  2. Frequently caused by prolonged exposure to glucocorticoid medication.

3. Signs and symptoms
    i. Weight gain
    ii. "Moon-faced" appearance
    iii. Fatty upper back ("buffalo hump")
    iv. Delayed wound healing
    v. Facial hair on women
    vi. Mood swings
4. Management
    i. General management of ALS patients (Patient Assessment chapter).

F. Addison's disease
   1. Adrenal disorder caused by adrenal insufficiency.
   2. Adrenals fail to produce adequate hormones.
   3. Signs and symptoms
       i. Progressive weakness, fatigue
       ii. Decreased appetite, weight loss
       iii. Hyperpigmentation of skin
       iv. Vomiting, diarrhea
       v. Cardiac dysrhythmias, circulator collapse
   4. Management
       i. General management of ALS patients (Patient Assessment chapter).
       ii. Administer dextrose if patient is hypoglycemic.
       iii. 12-lead ECG if evidence of dysrhythmias.
       iv. Aggressive fluid resuscitation.
       v. Rapid transport.

Chapter 10

REVIEW QUESTIONS
(Answers on pg. 417.)

1. Your diabetic patient presents with deep, rapid respirations and decreased LOC. You should suspect:

    A. hypoglycemia.

    B. DKA.

    C. HHNC.

    D. insulin shock.

2. Which endocrine gland stimulates the fight or flight response?

    A. adrenals

    B. thyroid

    C. hypothalamus

    D. pituitary

3. Your diabetic patient has a rapid deterioration in consciousness. You should suspect:

    A. hyperglycemia.

    B. DKA.

    C. HHNC.

    D. insulin shock.

4. Your patient presents with dull flank pain that gets worse when supine. The patient also has jaundice, fever, and nausea. Which of the following is most likely?

    A. Graves' disease

    B. thyroid storm

    C. pancreatitis

    D. appendicitis

5. Which of the following is an adrenal disorder caused by hyperadrenalism and prolonged use of glucocorticoid medication?

   A. Cushing's syndrome

   B. myxedema

   C. thyroid storm

   D. Addison's disease

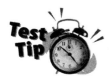

"I Will Pass" Checklist:

1. Did you previously pass the NREMT exam at the EMT or AEMT level?
2. Are you fully committed to becoming a paramedic?
3. Have you completed a CoAEMSP-accredited paramedic education program?
4. Are you willing to dedicate some focused study time **every day**?

If you answered YES to these questions, odds are strongly in your favor! This book is designed to help you with step 4. You can do this!

Anaphylaxis

Chapter 11

I. TERMS TO KNOW

A. **Anaphylactoid reaction:** Reactions that present like anaphylaxis, but are not IgE mediated.

B. **Anaphylaxis:** Life-threatening allergic reaction. Unlike anaphylactoid reactions, anaphylaxis requires the patient to be sensitized, and mediated through IgE antibodies.

C. **Antibodies:** Immune cells produced by body to attack invading substances.

D. **Antigen:** Any substance that can produce an immune response.

E. **Urticaria:** Hives (red, raised bumps across the body).

II. ANATOMY & PHYSIOLOGY REVIEW

Note: See "Circulatory System" and "Respiratory System" in the online Anatomy & Physiology Review at *www.rea.com/paramedic*.

III. COMMON CAUSES OF ANAPHYLAXIS

A. Insects (bees, wasps)

B. Plants

C. Foods (nuts, eggs, shellfish, milk, wheat, soy)

Chapter 11

D. Medications (antibiotics, aspirin, dextran)

E. Blood products

F. Radiographic contrast media

G. *Note:* Patients with asthma are at higher risk of severe allergic reaction.

 IV. SIGNS AND SYMPTOMS OF ANAPHYLAXIS

A. *Note:* Typically, signs and symptoms develop within 1 minute of exposure but in rare cases, may be delayed. Typically, the faster the onset, the worse the reaction.

B. Central nervous system
   1. Sense of impending doom
   2. Altered/decreased level of consciousness
   3. Seizures

C. Respiratory
   1. Dyspnea
   2. Wheezing, stridor
   3. Pulmonary edema
   4. Laryngospasm, bronchospasm

D. Cardiovascular
   1. Tachycardia
   2. Hypotension

E. Gastrointestinal
   1. Nausea, vomiting, abdominal cramps
   2. Occurs most often due to food-induced anaphylaxis

F. Skin

1. Flushed

2. Urticaria (hives)

3. Swelling

4. Diaphoresis

5. Cyanosis

6. *Note:* Many patients in anaphylactic shock do not present with urticaria or swelling (especially children).

V. BIPHASIC ANAPHYLAXIS

A. Biphasic anaphylaxis can occur up to 72 hours after the initial attack, without re-exposure to an allergen.

B. The incidence of biphasic anaphylaxis is unclear; however, it may occur in up to 20% of anaphylaxis cases.

VI. MANAGEMENT OF ANAPHYLAXIS

A. Ensure scene safety, e.g., chemicals, bees, etc.

B. Epinephrine administration intramuscular (IM) or intravenous (IV) per local protocol. *Note:* Do not delay. Epinephrine is the primary treatment for anaphylaxis.

C. Aggressive management of airway, breathing, circulation

1. High-flow oxygen.

2. Advanced airway as indicated.

3. Ventilatory support as indicated.

4. Treat for shock.

5. Aggressive isotonic IV fluid resuscitation.

6. Rapid transport.

Chapter 11

   D. Bronchodilator medications (albuterol and/or ipratropium) for bronchospasm
      1. *Note:* Can be administered via small volume nebulizer or in-line during bag-valve-mask ventilation.
   E. Consider antihistamines, such as diphenhydramine, per local protocol.
      1. *Note:* Epinephrine **first** for life-threatening anaphylaxis.
   F. There is no proven benefit of steroid administration for anaphylaxis.
   G. Consider glucagon for patients unresponsive to epinephrine.
      1. *Note:* Glucagon may be effective for anaphylactic patients on beta-blockers. Use in addition to (not instead of) epinephrine. Glucagon may also help reverse bronchospasm.
      2. Glucagon can reverse bronchospasm and hypotension in patients on beta-blockers by bypassing beta-adrenergic receptors.

VII. TRANSPLANT-RELATED PROBLEMS

   A. Infection
   B. Rejection
   C. Drug toxicity

REVIEW QUESTIONS
(Answers on pg. 418.)

1. Death from anaphylactic shock is typically the result of:
   A. infection.
   B. circulatory failure.
   C. massive systemic vasoconstriction.
   D. systemic urticaria.

2. Which of the following is **NOT** a common cause of anaphylaxis?

   A. insects

   B. plants

   C. radiographic contrast media

   D. latex

3. Which of the following is the primary treatment for anaphylaxis?

   A. oxygen

   B. albuterol

   C. epinephrine

   D. diphenhydramine

4. Which of the following may help treat anaphylaxis in patients on beta-blockers who are unresponsive to epinephrine?

   A. glucagon

   B. glucocorticoids

   C. dextrose

   D. calcium chloride

5. Nausea, vomiting, and diarrhea are most common in patients with:

   A. medication-induced anaphylaxis.

   B. food-induced anaphylaxis.

   C. exercise-induced anaphylaxis.

   D. insect-induced anaphylaxis.

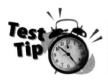

Once you complete your paramedic education program, develop your study plan and take the certification exam within 30 days (sooner if possible). Your odds of passing the test go down the longer you wait.

PART V
MEDICAL EMERGENCIES
(Part 2)

Gastrointestinal/ Genitourinary

I. TERMS TO KNOW

A. **Cullen's sign:** Bruising around the umbilicus. Possible sign on acute pancreatitis or retroperitoneal hemorrhage.

B. **Peritonitis:** Inflammation of the peritoneum.

C. **Referred pain:** Pain felt somewhere other than where it originates.

D. **Somatic pain:** Sharp, localized pain.

E. **Visceral pain:** Vague, diffuse, dull, cramp-like pain.

II. ANATOMY & PHYSIOLOGY REVIEW

Note: See "Abdominal Cavity" in the online Anatomy & Physiology Review at *www.rea.com/paramedic*.

III. UPPER GI CONDITIONS

A. Abdominal aortic aneurysm: See Cardiology & Resuscitation chapter.

B. Esophageal varices
   1. Swollen veins in the esophagus.
   2. Usually due to liver damage from alcohol abuse.
   3. Ruptured esophageal varices has high mortality rate due to massive hemorrhage, shock.

4. Management
    i. General management of advanced life support (ALS) patients (Patient Assessment chapter).
        ➤ Aggressive airway management likely necessary.
        ➤ Aggressive fluid resuscitation for shock.
        ➤ Consider antiemetics, such as ondansetron (Zofran).
        ➤ Rapid transport.

C. Gastroenteritis
    1. Inflammation of stomach and intestine with vomiting and/or diarrhea.
        i. *Note:* Gastritis is inflammation of the stomach only.
    2. Severe diarrhea can lead to hypovolemic shock.
        i. Pediatrics and elderly at increased risk of hypovolemic shock.
    3. Management
        i. Strictly follow Standard Precautions to reduce exposure risk.
        ii. General management of ALS patients (Patient Assessment chapter).
        iii. Protect airway to reduce risk of aspiration.
        iv. Aggressive fluid resuscitation for shock.
        v. Transport.

D. Peptic ulcer
    1. Erosion somewhere along the GI tract due to gastric acid.
    2. Signs and symptoms
        i. Often (not always) males over age 50, possibly under high stress
        ii. Often history of heavy use of aspirin, ibuprofen, alcohol, nicotine
        iii. Increased pain after eating
    3. Management
        i. General management of ALS patients (Patient Assessment chapter).

Gastrointestinal/Genitourinary

IV. LOWER GI CONDITIONS

A. Ulcerative colitis

1. Inflammatory bowel disorder of the large intestine, usually beginning between the ages of 15–30 years.

2. Creates chronic, linear ulcers in colon.

3. Signs and symptoms

   i. Acute abdominal cramping

   ii. Nausea & vomiting (N&V)

   iii. Bloody diarrhea or stool with mucus

   iv. Possible hypovolemic shock (severe cases)

4. Management

   i. General management of ALS patients (Patient Assessment chapter).

   ii. Observe for signs and symptoms of shock.

   iii. Consider antiemetics.

   iv. Transport.

B. Crohn's disease

1. Inflammatory bowel disorder.

2. Can occur anywhere from mouth to rectum.

3. Most common among white females, possibly under high stress.

4. Signs and symptoms

   i. GI bleeding

   ii. Weight loss

   iii. Diffuse abdominal pain

   iv. N&V

   v. Diarrhea

   vi. Fever

5. Management

   i. General management of ALS patients (Patient Assessment chapter).

Chapter 12

C. Diverticulitis
1. Inflammation or infection of small pouches along wall of intestine.
2. Signs and symptoms
   i. Abdominal pain, usually left lower quadrant
   ii. Fever
   iii. N&V
   iv. Hematochezia
3. Management
   i. General management of ALS patients (Patient Assessment chapter).

D. Irritable bowel syndrome
1. Aka spastic colon.
2. Can occur due to stress, after bacterial infection, or parasitic infection of the intestines.
3. Signs and symptoms
   i. Abdominal distention
   ii. Abdominal pain and cramping
   iii. Constipation
   iv. Constipation or diarrhea
   v. Increased gas
   vi. Loss of appetite
   vii. Nausea
4. Management
   i. General management of ALS patients (Patient Assessment chapter).

E. Bowel obstruction
1. Can be life-threatening.
2. Frequently caused by abdominal adhesions or malignancies.

3. Signs and symptoms
   i. Visceral abdominal pain and tenderness
   ii. Signs and symptoms of shock
4. Management
   i. General management of ALS patients (Patient Assessment chapter).

F. Appendicitis
  1. Most common surgical emergency encountered by EMS.
  2. Usually occurs between age 10 and 30.
  3. Rupture leads to peritonitis.
  4. Signs and symptoms
     i. Diffuse periumbilical abdominal pain (early)
     ii. N&V
     iii. Loss of appetite
     iv. Right lower quadrant pain or rebound tenderness (late)
     v. *Note:* Pain often becomes diffuse again after rupture.
  5. Management
     i. General management of ALS patients (Patient Assessment chapter).
     ii. Transport for diagnostic computed tomography.

G. Cholecystitis
  1. Inflammation of the gall bladder.
  2. Signs and symptoms
     i. Right upper quadrant abdominal pain
     ii. Referred pain to right shoulder
     iii. N&V
  3. Management
     i. General management of ALS patients (Patient Assessment chapter).
     ii. Consider analgesic meds per local protocol.

Chapter 12

H. Pancreatitis
   1. Inflammation of the pancreas. Gallstones and alcohol abuse account for 80% of cases.
   2. Signs and symptoms
      i. Severe abdominal pain
      ii. N&V
      iii. Cullen's sign
      iv. Possible signs and symptoms of shock
   3. Management
      i. General management of ALS patients (Patient Assessment chapter).
      ii. Fluid resuscitation for shock.

I. Hepatitis
   1. Inflammation of the liver.
   2. High mortality rate.
   3. Often associated with alcohol abuse.
   4. Signs and symptoms
      i. Right upper quadrant abdominal tenderness
      ii. Loss of appetite
      iii. Jaundice
      iv. N&V
      v. Weakness
   5. Management
      i. General management of ALS patients (Patient Assessment chapter).
      ii. Follow standard precautions and use appropriate personal protective equipment (PPE) when caring for patients with a suspected infection, such as hepatitis.

Gastrointestinal/Genitourinary

 V. GENITOURINARY CONDITIONS

  A. Acute renal failure

    1. Pathophysiology

        i. Sudden and dangerous (but potentially reversible) drop in urinary output.

        ii. Kidneys acutely unable to filter waste products from blood.

        iii. Typically occurs in seriously ill or injured patients.

        iv. High mortality rate (about 50%).

    2. Signs and symptoms

        i. Oliguria: Reduced urinary output

        ii. Anuria: No urinary output

        iii. History of shock, myocardial infarction, congestive heart failure, or sepsis

        iv. Painful bladder fullness

        v. Edema

    3. Management

        i. General management of ALS patients (Patient Assessment chapter).

        ii. Treat for shock as indicated.

        iii. High-priority transport.

  B. Chronic renal failure

    1. Pathophysiology

        i. Inadequate kidney function due to irreversible kidney damage.

        ii. Often due to diabetes or hypertension.

        iii. End-stage renal failure requires dialysis or kidney transplant.

            ➤ Risks of dialysis

                — Electrolyte imbalance

                — Hypotension

                — Hemorrhage

                — Infection

2. Signs and symptoms
    i. Altered level of consciousness
    ii. Edema
    iii. History of diabetes or hypertension
3. Management
    i. See management of acute renal failure.

C. Renal calculi (kidney stones)
1. Mass of calcium compounds in kidneys.
2. Signs and symptoms
    i. Severe flank or groin pain
    ii. N&V
    iii. Hematuria
    iv. Painful urination and decreased or blocked urinary output
    v. Fever
    vi. Pale, clammy
3. Management
    i. General management of ALS patients (Patient Assessment chapter).
    ii. Analgesic and antiemetic medications per local protocol.
    iii. Transport.

D. Urinary tract infection (UTI)
1. Pathophysiology: More common in females, paraplegics, and sexually active persons.
2. Signs and symptoms
    i. Painful urination
    ii. Frequent urination
    iii. Difficulty urinating
    iv. Foul odor in urine
    v. History of previous UTIs

vi. Fever

vii. Back or flank pain, lower abdominal pain

3. Management

 i. General management of ALS patients (Patient Assessment chapter).

REVIEW QUESTIONS
(Answers on pg. 418.)

1. Bruising around the umbilicus is known as:

    A. circumferential edema.

    B. Cullen's sign.

    C. melena.

    D. angioedema.

2. Which of the following is usually due to liver damage from alcohol abuse?

    A. cholecystitis

    B. pulmonary hypertension

    C. gastroenteritis

    D. esophageal varices

3. Your patient is a 55-year-old male who presents with increased abdominal pain after eating. He has a history of heavy aspirin, ibuprofen, and nicotine use. Which of the following is most likely?

    A. abdominal aortic aneurysm

    B. diverticulitis

    C. peptic ulcer

    D. appendicitis

Chapter 12

4. Your patient is in his mid-20's and complains of acute abdominal cramping, nausea and vomiting, and bloody diarrhea with mucus. Which of the following conditions is most likely?

   A. ulcerative colitis

   B. gastroenteritis

   C. Crohn's disease

   D. appendicitis

5. Your patient is a 16-year-old male complaining of abdominal pain. The patient states the pain was initially diffuse but is now localized to the right lower quadrant. You should suspect:

   A. irritable bowel syndrome.

   B. appendicitis.

   C. pancreatitis.

   D. hepatitis.

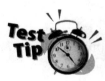

Consider creating a brief (2–3 sentences) pathophysiology flashcard for common medical emergencies and traumatic injuries covered in this book.

Sample Patho Card Front:

Describe the pathophysiology of shock

Sample Patho Card Back:

Shock is inadequate tissue perfusion due to a pump (heart), pipe (vessels), or fluid (blood volume) problem.

Chapter 13

Toxicology

I. TERMS TO KNOW

A. **Miosis:** Pupillary constriction (may be caused by narcotic overdose or cholinergic poisoning).

B. **Mydriasis:** Pupillary dilation (may be caused by stimulants or adrenergic poisoning).

C. **Toxidromes:** Group of signs and symptoms for a specific group of toxins, e.g., stimulants, narcotics, etc.

II. EPIDEMIOLOGY

A. Most accidental poisonings involve children but are less likely fatal.

B. Adult poisoning and overdoses are less common, but more likely fatal.

C. Most suicide attempts involve a drug overdose.

III. ROUTES OF EXPOSURE

A. Ingestion

B. Inhalation

C. Injection

D. Surface absorption

Chapter 13

 IV. GENERAL MANAGEMENT OF TOXICOLOGIC EMERGENCY

    A. High index of suspicion for scene safety hazards.

    B. Remove from source of exposure as indicated.

    C. General management of advanced life support (ALS) patients (Patient Assessment chapter).

    D. Attempt to identify specific toxin(s).

    E. Consider decontamination interventions per local protocol.

    F. Consider specific antidotes if available.

    G. Contact Poison Control Center for additional information as indicated: (800) 222-1222.

 V. DECONTAMINATION PROCEDURES

    A. External decontamination
        1. Remove contaminated clothing.
        2. Remove stingers.
        3. Decontamination shower.

    B. Internal decontamination
        1. Intended to reduce absorption of ingested toxins.
        2. *Note:* These methods have diminished application in the prehospital setting in many EMS systems.
            i. Syrup of ipecac: **Not** used in prehospital setting any longer.
            ii. Gastric lavage: Limited benefit and high risk of complications.
            iii. Activated charcoal: Most commonly used prehospital method of internal decontamination of ingested toxins.

VI. COMMON TOXIDROMES

A. Cholinergics (see Specific Toxins section)

B. Sympathomimetics/stimulants (see Specific Toxins section)

C. Barbiturates/hypnotics (see Specific Toxins section)

D. Hallucinogens (see Specific Toxins section)

E. Opiates (see Specific Toxins section)

F. Anticholinergics
   1. Caused by numerous medications, plants, chemicals.
   2. Signs and symptoms
      i. "hot as Hades"
      ii. "blind as a bat"
      iii. "dry as a bone"
      iv. "red as a beet"
      v. "mad as a hatter"

G. Marijuana and cannabis
   1. Can be smoked or consumed.
   2. Can produce euphoria, relaxation, heightened sensory perception, laughter, increased appetite.

H. Huffing agents
   1. Examples: metallic paint, paint thinner, Super Glue
   2. Can cause cardiovascular collapse, ventricular dysrhythmias, seizures.

Chapter 13

SPECIFIC TOXINS

A. Carbon monoxide
1. Signs and symptoms
   i. SpCO above 5% in nonsmokers and 10% in smokers
   ii. Fatigue
   iii. Headache
   iv. Dizziness
   v. Nausea & vomiting (N&V)
   vi. Confusion
   vii. Coma
   viii. Dyspnea
   ix. Chest pain
   x. Cardiac dysrhythmias
   xi. Seizures
2. Management
   i. Remove patient from source of CO as safety permits.
   ii. General management of ALS patients.
   iii. **Must** administer high-concentration oxygen.
   iv. Consider continuous positive airway pressure (CPAP).
   v. Transport to hyperbaric chamber, per local protocol.

B. Cyanide
1. Signs and symptoms
   i. Headache
   ii. Confusion
   iii. Patient may detect bitter almond smell
   iv. Pulmonary edema
   v. Seizures
   vi. Coma

2. Management
    i. Remove from source as safety permits.
    ii. Cyanide ingestion will react with stomach acid, generating hydrogen cyanide gas (maximize air circulation in ambulance).
    iii. High-concentration oxygen via nonrebreather, CPAP, or bag-valve-mask (do not rely on accuracy of pulse oximetry).
    iv. Administer hydroxocobalamin (Cyano-Kit) or sodium thiosulfate.
        ➤ Classic cyanide antidote kits of amyl nitrite and sodium nitrite no longer available.
        ➤ Hydroxocobalamin will turn skin, tears, and urine red. This does not indicate an allergic reaction.

> ➤ *Remember:* Know the signs and symptoms of exposure to pesticides and nerve agents. Use the SLUDGEM or DUMBELS acronym.

C. Cholinergics/organophosphates/nerve agents
    1. Present in pesticides and various nerve agents.
    2. Causes (potentially massive) overstimulation of cholinergic (parasympathetic) nervous system.
    3. Signs and symptoms (SLUDGEM and DUMBELS)
        i. SLUDGEM mnemonic
            ➤ Salivation, seizures
            ➤ Lacrimation (excessive tearing)
            ➤ Urination
            ➤ Defecation
            ➤ Gastric upset
            ➤ Emesis
            ➤ Miosis (pupillary constriction)
        ii. DUMBELS mnemonic
            ➤ Diarrhea
            ➤ Urination

- Miosis
- Bradycardia, bronchospasm
- Emesis
- Lacrimation
- Seizures, salivation

    4. Management
- i. External decontamination as indicated.
- ii. General management of ALS patients.
- iii. Atropine 2–5 mg IM/IV/IO q 3–5 minutes as indicated.
- iv. Pralidoxime (2-Pam) per local protocol.
- v. *Note:* Atropine and pralidoxime can be administered together in an autoinjector called DuoDote (single IM injection) or MARK 1 (two IM injections).

D. Cardiac medications
1. Signs and symptoms
   - i. Cardiac dysrhythmias
   - ii. Hypotension
   - iii. N&V
   - iv. Pulmonary edema
2. Management
   - i. General management of ALS patients (Patient Assessment chapter).
   - ii. Be prepared to initiate external cardiac pacing.
   - iii. Consider IV calcium for calcium channel blocker overdose.
   - iv. Consider glucagon for beta-blocker overdose.

E. Caustics (acids and alkalis)
1. Present in many household cleaners.
2. Signs and symptoms
   - i. Burns
   - ii. Dyspnea

iii. Stridor

iv. N&V

v. Hemorrhage

vi. Shock

3. Management

   i. General management of ALS patients (Patient Assessment chapter).

   ii. *Note:* Activated charcoal is **not** indicated.

F. Hydrocarbons

1. Found in kerosene, turpentine, mineral oil, lubricants, paint, glue, etc.

2. Signs and symptoms

   i. Burns

   ii. Dyspnea

   iii. Wheezing

   iv. Headache

   v. Dizziness

   vi. Cardiac dysrhythmias

3. Management

   i. General management of ALS patients (Patient Assessment chapter).

   ii. *Note:* Most hydrocarbon exposures are not serious if asymptomatic.

G. Cyclic antidepressants

1. Not as widely used now due to narrow therapeutic window. Includes amitriptyline (Elavil), doxepin, amoxapine, nortriptyline.

2. Signs and symptoms

   i. Blurred vision

   ii. Confusion

   iii. Respiratory depression

   iv. Seizures

Chapter 13

      v. Tachycardia

      vi. Hypotension

      vii. Cardiac dysrhythmias (especially AV block, wide QRS tachycardias)

  3. Management

      i. General management of ALS patients (Patient Assessment chapter).

      ii. Continuous ECG monitoring (high risk of death due to dysrhythmias).

      iii. Consider IV sodium bicarbonate per local protocol.

H. Monoamine oxidase (MAO) Inhibitors

  1. Used to treat depression, obsessive-compulsive disorder. Not widely used any longer due to risks.

  2. Signs and symptoms

      i. Hypertension or hypotension

      ii. Bradycardia or tachycardia

      iii. Hyperthermia

      iv. Headache

      v. Restless, agitation

      vi. Coma

  3. Management

      i. General management of ALS patients (Patient Assessment chapter).

      ii. Benzodiazepines for seizures per local protocol.

I. Lithium

  1. Commonly used for treatment of bipolar disorder. Has a narrow therapeutic index.

  2. Signs and symptoms

      i. Confusion

      ii. Thirst

      iii. N&V

Toxicology

      iv. Tremors

      v. Bradycardia

      vi. Cardiac dysrhythmias

      vii. Seizures

      viii. Coma

   3. Management

      i. General management of ALS patients (Patient Assessment chapter).

      ii. *Note:* Activated charcoal is not indicated.

J. Aspirin

   1. Signs and symptoms

      i. Tachypnea

      ii. Hyperthermia

      iii. Altered level of consciousness (LOC)

      iv. Coma

      v. Cardiac dysrhythmias

      vi. N&V

      vii. Pulmonary edema

   2. Management

      i. General management of ALS patients (Patient Assessment chapter).

      ii. Consider activated charcoal per local protocol.

      iii. Consider IV fluid resuscitation for symptomatic patients.

K. Acetaminophen (Tylenol)

   1. Signs and symptoms

      i. Fatigue

      ii. N&V

      iii. Abdominal pain

      iv. Liver damage

Chapter 13

    2. Management

        i. General management of ALS patients (Patient Assessment chapter).

        ii. Transport for possible N-acetylcysteine (NAC) administration.

        iii. *Note:* Concomitant use of NAC and activated charcoal is **not** recommended.

  L. Food poisoning

    1. Signs and symptoms

        i. N&V

        ii. Diarrhea

        iii. Abdominal pain

    2. Management

        i. General management of ALS patients (Patient Assessment chapter).

        ii. Treat for hypovolemia as indicated.

        iii. Consider antiemetics.

VIII. COMMONLY ABUSED DRUGS

  A. Alcohol

    1. Signs and symptoms

        i. Central nervous system (CNS) depression

        ii. Slurred speech

        iii. Impaired judgment

        iv. Unsteady gait

        v. N&V

    2. Alcohol withdrawal syndrome

        i. High mortality rate from seizures, delirium tremens (DTs).

        ii. Can last up to 1 week.

        iii. Seizures possible first 24–36 hours.

        iv. DTs possible second to third day of withdrawal.

- Decreased LOC
- Hallucinations
- Tremors
- N&V

3. Management
    i. General management of ALS patients (Patient Assessment chapter).
    ii. Consider thiamine.
    iii. Consider dextrose for hypoglycemia.
    iv. Consider benzodiazepines for DTs to prevent seizures.
    v. Benzodiazepines for seizures.

B. Methyl alcohol
    1. Aka wood alcohol and methanol.
    2. Present in antifreeze, paints, paint remover, windshield washer fluid.
    3. Abused as a substitute for drinking alcohol (ethanol).
    4. Signs and symptoms (12–71 hours after ingestion)
        i. Altered LOC
        ii. N&V
        iii. Headache
        iv. Dizziness
        v. Abdominal pain
        vi. Blurred vision
        vii. Tachypnea
        viii. Bradycardia
        ix. Hypotension
        x. Coma
    5. Management
        i. General management of ALS patients (Patient Assessment chapter).

- ii. Be alert for hypoglycemia. Dextrose as indicated.
- iii. Activated charcoal **not** indicated.
- iv. Consult Poison Control for additional recommendations.

C. Ethylene glycol
1. Found in paint, antifreeze.
2. May be abused as substitute for drinking alcohol.
3. Signs and symptoms
   - i. CNS depression
   - ii. Intoxicated appearance
   - iii. N&V
   - iv. Seizures
   - v. Coma
   - vi. Hypertension or hypotension
   - vii. Pulmonary edema
   - viii. Acute renal failure
4. Management
   - i. Same as methyl alcohol.

D. Amphetamines and stimulants
1. Examples: Adderall, Ritalin, cocaine, methamphetamine, bath salts, Benzedrine
2. Signs and symptoms
   - i. Hyperactivity
   - ii. Hypertension/Tachycardia
   - iii. Mydriasis
   - iv. Psychosis
   - v. Seizures
3. Management
   - i. General management of ALS patients (Patient Assessment chapter).
   - ii. Benzodiazepines for seizures.

E. Barbiturates
   1. Examples: thiopental, phenobarbital
   2. Signs and symptoms
      i. Decreased LOC, coma
      ii. Slurred speech
      iii. Nystagmus
      iv. Hypotension
      v. Respiratory depression
   3. Management
      i. General management of ALS patients (Patient Assessment chapter).

F. Benzodiazepines
   1. Examples: Valium, Xanax, Ativan
   2. Signs and symptoms
      i. Altered LOC
      ii. Slurred speech
      iii. Cardiac dysrhythmias
   3. Management
      i. General management of ALS patients (Patient Assessment chapter).
      ii. Consider activated charcoal.

G. Cocaine
   1. Signs and symptoms
      i. Euphoria
      ii. Tachycardia
      iii. Cardiac dysrhythmias
      iv. Mydriasis
      v. Hyperactivity
      vi. Hypertension/chest pain

- vii. Anxiety
- viii. Seizures
2. Management
    - i. General management of ALS patients (Patient Assessment chapter).
    - ii. Benzodiazepines for seizures.

H. Hallucinogens
 1. Examples: ketamine, LSD, MDMA, PCP, peyote, psilocybin mushrooms
 2. Signs and symptoms
    - i. Psychosis
    - ii. Incoherent speech
    - iii. Altered perception
 3. Management
    - i. Heightened scene safety, especially with patients on PCP.
    - ii. General management of ALS patients (Patient Assessment chapter).

I. Opioids
 1. Examples: heroin, codeine, morphine, fentanyl, hydrocodone, oxycodone, OxyContin, Vicodin (some contain opiates and acetaminophen)
 2. Signs and symptoms
    - i. CNS/respiratory depression
    - ii. Miosis
    - iii. Hypotension
    - iv. Bradycardia
    - v. Coma
 3. Management
    - i. General management of ALS patients (Patient Assessment chapter).
    - ii. Aggressive ventilatory support.
    - iii. Naloxone.

J. Drugs used for sexual enhancement or sexual assault
  1. Ecstasy (MDMA)
     i. Stimulant drug; aka "E," "X," Molly.
     ii. Signs and symptoms
        ➤ Stimulant effects (hypertension, tachycardia)
        ➤ Euphoria
        ➤ Increased sexuality
        ➤ Altered perception of time and space
        ➤ Blurred vision/pupillary dilation
        ➤ Hyperthermia
        ➤ Seizures
     iii. Management
        ➤ General management of ALS patients (Patient Assessment chapter).
        ➤ Notify law enforcement and receiving hospital if sexual assault suspected.
  2. Rohypnol (flunitrazepam)
     i. Potent benzodiazepine; aka R2, Roofies, Rope.
     ii. Signs and symptoms
        ➤ CNS depression
        ➤ Sedation
        ➤ Amnesia
        ➤ Bradycardia
        ➤ Respiratory depression
        ➤ Coma
     iii. Management
        ➤ General management of ALS patients (Patient Assessment chapter).
        ➤ Notify law enforcement and receiving hospital if sexual assault suspected.

3. Gamma-hydroxybutyrate (GHB)
   i. Produces intoxication similar to alcohol; aka Liquid Ecstasy.
   ii. Signs and symptoms
      ➤ Euphoria
      ➤ Reduced inhibition
      ➤ Amnesia
      ➤ Respiratory depression
      ➤ Coma
   iii. Management
      ➤ General management of ALS patients (Patient Assessment chapter).
      ➤ Notify law enforcement and receiving hospital if sexual assault suspected.
4. Ketamine
   i. Also called K, Special K, Vitamin K.
   ii. Potent anesthetic, similar to LSD.
   iii. Causes hallucinations, amnesia, dissociative state.

SPECIAL PATIENTS

A. Pediatrics
   1. Lithium button/coin batteries
      i. Extremely dangerous when ingested (pediatric patients under age 6 at highest risk).
      ii. Can generate an electrical current when in contact with body fluid, causing severe burns.
      iii. Can burn through esophagus in 2 hours.
   2. Magnets
      i. Ingestion of multiple high-power magnets is extremely dangerous.
      ii. Magnetic attraction can cause tissue ischemia, pressure necrosis, tissue rupture, hemorrhage, and sepsis.

3. E-cigarettes

   i. Liquid nicotine ingestion (less than half a teaspoon) can be fatal in pediatric patients.

   ii. Signs and symptoms include diaphoresis, dizziness, vomiting, tachycardia.

REVIEW QUESTIONS
(Answers on pg. 419.)

1. Which of the following toxidromes causes patients to be hot, dry, blind, and flushed?

   A. anticholinergics

   B. cholinergics

   C. opioids

   D. hallucinogens

2. Which of the following toxidromes presents with diarrhea, urination, miosis, bradycardia, emesis, lacrimation, and seizures?

   A. anticholinergics

   B. opioids

   C. cholinergics

   D. hallucinogens

3. Your patient has been exposed to a potentially deadly nerve agent. Which of the following is indicated?

   A. epinephrine 1 mg

   B. diphenhydramine 50 mg

   C. midazolam 2 mg

   D. atropine 2 mg

Chapter 13

4. Which of the following is contraindicated for patients that have ingested strong acids or alkalis?

   A. oxygen

   B. IV access

   C. rapid transport

   D. activated charcoal

5. Your patient presents with psychosis, incoherent speech, and altered perceptions of reality. You should suspect:

   A. cocaine overdose.

   B. MDMA overdose.

   C. Valium overdose.

   D. Tylenol overdose.

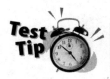

Test Tip Everyone will feel like the certification exam is challenging. You will intentionally be given questions designed to test the limits of your knowledge. Don't let this stress you out or distract you! Stay calm and focused, and trust your abilities.

Hematology and Infectious Disease

I. TERMS TO KNOW

A. **Anemias:** Inadequate red blood cells (RBCs). Can be chronic or acute. Can be caused by inadequate RBC production, RBC destruction, hemorrhage, or dilution of RBCs.

B. **Disseminated intravascular coagulation:** Abnormal blood clotting throughout the body.

C. **Hemophilia:** Clotting disorder.

D. **MRSA:** Drug-resistant bacterial infection.

E. **Plasma:** Fluid component of blood.

II. ANATOMY & PHYSIOLOGY REVIEW

Note: See "Circulatory System" in the online Anatomy & Physiology Review at *www.rea.com/paramedic*.

III. HEMATOLOGICAL DISORDERS

A. Transfusion reactions

　1. Causes

　　i. Hemolytic reaction

　　ii. Febrile reaction

　　iii. Allergic reaction

Chapter 14

        iv. Lung injury
        v. Circulatory overload
        vi. Infection
    2. Signs and symptoms
        i. Hyperventilation
        ii. Tachycardia
        iii. Sense of impending doom
        iv. Flushing and hives
        v. Fever
        vi. Chest pain
        vii. Dyspnea
        viii. Flank pain
    3. Management
        i. Stop blood transfusion.
        ii. Change all IV tubings.
        iii. IV normal saline or lactated Ringer's.
        iv. Consider diuretics, vasopressors, antihistamines per local protocol.

B. Sickle cell disease (sickle cell anemia)
    1. Sickle cell disease is one form of anemia. Anemias are caused by inadequate RBCs. Anemias can be chronic or acute. Can be caused by inadequate RBC production, RBC destruction, hemorrhage, or dilution of RBCs.
    2. Pathophysiology of sickle cell disease
        i. Inherited chronic anemia primarily affecting people of African, Mediterranean, and Middle Eastern descent.
        ii. Causes creation and premature destruction of abnormal (sickle-shaped) RBCs.
        iii. Sludging of blood causes obstruction of microvasculature and vaso-occlusive crisis.
        iv. Increased risk of renal failure, stroke, sepsis.

3. Signs and symptoms
    i. Musculoskeletal pain
    ii. Abdominal pain
    iii. Priapism
4. Management
    i. General management of advanced life support (ALS) patients (Patient Assessment chapter).
    ii. Analgesic meds per local protocol.

C. Leukemia
   1. Cancer of the body's blood-forming tissues.
   2. Signs and symptoms
       i. Weakness
       ii. Increased risk of anemia, hemorrhage
       iii. Fever
       iv. Weight loss
   3. Management
       i. General management of ALS patients (Patient Assessment chapter).

D. Lymphomas
   1. Cancer of lymphatic system. Includes Hodgkin's lymphoma and non-Hodgkin's lymphoma.
   2. Signs and symptoms
       i. Swelling of lymph nodes
       ii. Fever
       iii. Night sweats
       iv. Fatigue
       v. Weight loss
   3. Management
       i. General management of ALS patients (Patient Assessment chapter).

- E. Hemophilia
    1. Clotting disorder causing poor bleeding control.
    2. Signs and symptoms
        i. Extensive bruising
        ii. Bleeding that is difficult to control
        iii. Look for medic alert bracelet
    3. Management
        i. General management of ALS patients (Patient Assessment chapter).
- F. Disseminated intravascular coagulation (DIC)
    1. Pathophysiology
        i. Coagulation disorder due to deficiency of clotting factors.
        ii. Often due to sepsis, hypovolemic shock, obstetrical complications, cancers, hemolytic transfusion reactions.
    2. Signs and symptoms
        i. Bleeding
        ii. Hypotension
        iii. Shock
    3. Management
        i. General management of ALS patients (Patient Assessment chapter).
- G. Multiple myeloma
    1. Cancer of plasma cells.
    2. Signs and symptoms
        i. Back or rib pain
        ii. Fatigue
        iii. Pathological fractures
        iv. Hemorrhage
    3. Management
        i. General management of ALS patients (Patient Assessment chapter).

Hematology and Infectious Disease

IV. INFECTIOUS DISEASES

A. Pathophysiology

1. Bacterial infections

   i. Typically respond to antibiotics.

   ii. Example: strep throat, urinary tract infection (UTI), food poisoning, gonorrhea, bacterial meningitis.

2. Viral infections

   i. Resistant to antibiotics.

   ii. Example: COVID-19, influenza, common cold, varicella, HIV, viral meningitis.

3. Epidemic and pandemic

   i. Epidemic: Widespread occurrence of disease in a community at a particular time.

   ii. Pandemic: Outbreak of disease across several countries or continents.

B. Sepsis red flags

1. You should suspect sepsis if your patient presents with an obvious or suspected infection **and** any **two** of the following criteria:

   i. Tachypnea (above about 20 breaths per minute).

   ii. Fever (about 100.4°F or above).

   iii. Pulse rate above about 90 per minute.

2. Follow local protocols regarding sepsis management and receiving hospital notification (sepsis alert).

C. HIV/AIDS

1. Blood-borne pathogen with no cure or vaccine.

2. Not highly contagious.

3. Patients with HIV/AIDS require compassionate, nonjudgmental supportive care.

4. If exposed, immediately contact Infection Control Officer or seek care for possible postexposure therapy (some therapies must be initiated within hours).

|207

Chapter 14

D. Hepatitis
1. There are at least five different types of hepatitis. Follow general management of ALS patient guidelines (Patient Assessment chapter).
2. Hepatitis A
   i. Transmitted by fecal-oral route.
   ii. Often asymptomatic and not often life-threatening.
   iii. Vaccine available.
3. Hepatitis B
   i. Highly contagious blood-borne pathogen with substantial risk to EMS personnel.
   ii. Up to 40% infection rate following contaminated needle stick.
   iii. Can lead to hepatitis, cirrhosis, liver cancer.
   iv. Patients may be asymptomatic.
   v. Vaccine available.
4. Hepatitis C
   i. Blood-borne, often due to IV drug abuse, sexual contact, or blood transfusion prior to 1992.
   ii. Patients may be asymptomatic for years.
   iii. Disease accelerated in older patients or those consuming alcohol.
   iv. Hepatitis C is now curable.

E. Tuberculosis (TB)
1. Highly contagious but treatable airborne bacterial infection.
2. Signs and symptoms
   i. Fatigue
   ii. Fever and night sweats
   iii. Chills
   iv. Chronic cough and hemoptysis
   v. Weight loss

3. Management
    i. High index of suspicion based on signs and symptoms.
    ii. Can remain dormant for years.
    iii. Use approved N95 or high-efficiency particulate air (HEPA) mask.
    iv. General management of ALS patients (Patient Assessment chapter).

F. Pneumonia
    1. Lung inflammation due to bacterial or viral infection.
    2. High-risk patients/conditions
        i. Immunosuppressed
        ii. Sickle cell disease
        iii. Organ transplant
        iv. Cancer
        v. Ventilator-dependent
        vi. Elderly
        vii. Low-birth-weight neonates
        viii. Chronic lung disease
        ix. Aspiration
    3. Signs and symptoms
        i. Weakness
        ii. Fever
        iii. Chills
        iv. Altered level of consciousness (LOC)
        v. Dyspnea
        vi. Chest pain (worsened on inspiration)
        vii. Persistent, productive cough
        viii. Fever, tachypnea, retractions in pediatrics
        ix. *Note:* Consider pneumonia for any patient with fever and tachypnea.

Chapter 14

    4. Management
- i. Wear N95 or HEPA mask as indicated.
- ii. General management of ALS patients (Patient Assessment chapter).
- iii. Consider continuous positive airway pressure.

G. Meningitis
1. Bacterial or viral infection causing inflammation of the meninges.
   - i. *Note:* Bacterial meningitis can be acutely life-threatening. Viral meningitis is typically less severe.
2. Signs and symptoms
   - i. Weakness
   - ii. Decreased LOC
   - iii. Fever
   - iv. Chills
   - v. Headache
   - vi. Nuchal rigidity
   - vii. Nausea & vomiting (N&V)
   - viii. Photophobia
   - ix. Seizures
   - x. Brudzinski's sign: Flexion of neck causes flexion of hips and knees
   - xi. Kernig's sign: Inability to fully extend knee with hips flexed
3. Management
   - i. Use mask and place mask on patient when possible.
   - ii. Meningococcal vaccines.
   - iii. Seek medical attention for possible postexposure prophylaxis.
   - iv. General management of ALS patients (Patient Assessment chapter).

H. Measles, mumps, rubella (MMR)
1. All three are airborne diseases.

2. MMR vaccine is about 99% effective and generally required for healthcare workers.
3. Signs and symptoms
    i. Cold-like symptoms
    ii. Rash
    iii. Fever
4. Management
    i. Wear N95 or HEPA mask as indicated. Place mask on patient too, when able.
    ii. General management of ALS patients (Patient Assessment chapter).

I. Respiratory syncytial virus (RSV)
    1. Highly infectious, potentially fatal respiratory infection, especially in infants and children.
    2. Occurrences most common during winter.
    3. Signs and symptoms
        i. Cold-like symptoms (usually no more than this in adults)
        ii. Wheezes
        iii. Tachypnea
        iv. Respiratory distress
        v. *Note:* Assume an infant with wheezing during winter months has RSV until proven otherwise.
    4. Management
        i. Wear N95 or HEPA mask as indicated.
        ii. General management of ALS patients (Patient Assessment chapter).

J. Pertussis (whooping cough)
    1. Signs and symptoms
        i. Cold-like symptoms
        ii. Fever
        iii. Severe, violent cough

Chapter 14

2. Management
    i. General management of ALS patients (Patient Assessment chapter).

K. Laryngotracheobronchitis (croup)
    1. Common viral respiratory infection (especially in children 3 and under).
    2. **Not** generally life-threatening (complete airway obstruction from croup is rare).
    3. Signs and symptoms
        i. Acute-onset respiratory distress
        ii. Stridor
        iii. "Barking seal" or tight, low-pitched cough

L. Epiglottitis
    1. Inflammation of the epiglottis that can lead to complete airway obstruction.
    2. Signs and symptoms
        i. Acute onset without recent history of cold-like symptoms
            ➤ Difficulty speaking
            ➤ Difficulty swallowing
            ➤ Drooling
            ➤ Dyspnea
            ➤ Stridor
            ➤ Sore throat
            ➤ Fever
    3. Management
        i. Avoid further distressing or upsetting child due to risk of airway obstruction.
        ii. General management of ALS patients (Patient Assessment chapter).
        iii. In the event of complete or nearly complete airway obstruction, positive pressure ventilation may be difficult, but is usually possible.

M. Drug-resistant bacterial infections

1. Bacteria and other microorganisms resistant to antibiotics. A major concern of overuse of antibiotics.
2. Examples
    i. MRSA: methicillin-resistant *Staphylococcus aureus*.
    ii. VRSA: vancomycin-resistant *Staphylococcus aureus*.
    iii. VRE: vancomycin-resistant *Enterococcus*.

N. Rabies

1. A deadly virus spread to people from the saliva of infected animals.
2. Treatable with early postexposure treatment; generally fatal once symptomatic.
3. Clean wound and assume exposure risk anytime there is exposure to saliva of potentially infected animal.

V. SEXUALLY TRANSMITTED DISEASES (STDs)

A. Gonorrhea and chlamydia

1. Gonorrhea and chlamydia are different STDs, with similar signs and symptoms.
2. Signs and symptoms
    i. Painful urination
    ii. Urethral discharge
    iii. Fever
3. Management
    i. General management of ALS patients (Patient Assessment chapter).
    ii. Can lead to sepsis, meningitis, pelvic inflammatory disease, or sterility if untreated.

B. Syphilis

1. Signs and symptoms
    i. Lesions (can occur anywhere)
    ii. Rash

2. Management

   i. General management of ALS patients (Patient Assessment chapter).

VI. PRECAUTION LEVELS AND DISINFECTION

A. Standard precautions

1. Replaces "universal precautions" and "BSI [body substance isolation] precautions."

2. Precautions apply to all body substances except sweat.

3. Employers required to develop infection control protocols and provide the necessary equipment and training.

4. Employees required to complete mandatory training and follow written protocols.

5. Use appropriate personal protective equipment (PPE) whenever there is an expectation of exposure to infectious material. Minimum PPE includes gloves and eye protection.

6. Appropriate PPE always includes handwashing before and after gloves. Preferred method includes antimicrobial, alcohol-based foams or gels with vigorous scrubbing for at least 20 seconds.

7. Expanded PPE: Use disposable gown, mask, face shield for significant contact with any body fluid, e.g., childbirth, severe hemorrhaging.

B. Airborne precautions

1. Use HEPA mask or N95 respirator for suspected airborne/droplet disease exposure, e.g., TB, meningitis.

2. Use appropriate airborne PPE precautions with suspected or confirmed cases of TB, chicken pox, measles.

3. Place a mask on the patient when possible.

C. Contaminated waste

1. Sharps (needles, lancets, etc.) must be placed in designated puncture-proof container. Do **not** recap used sharps.

2. Contaminated waste should be disposed of in "biohazard" bags and properly disposed of.

Hematology and Infectious Disease

3. *Note:* Per CDC and OSHA guidelines, tears, sweat, saliva, stool, urine, vomit, and oral and nasal secretions pose a risk for transmission of HIV, hepatitis B, or hepatitis C **only** if they contain visible blood.

D. Disinfection levels
   1. Low-level disinfection
      i. Kills most bacteria and some viruses.
      ii. Use for routine cleaning and removal of visible body fluids.
   2. Intermediate-level disinfection
      i. Kills most bacteria and most viruses.
      ii. Use for all medical equipment that was in contact with patient's skin.
      iii. Can use 1:10 – 1:100 chlorine bleach–to–water solution or chemical germicide.
   3. High-level disinfection
      i. Kills almost all microorganisms.
      ii. Use for all reusable medical equipment that was in contact with patient's mucous membranes.
      iii. Immerse in chemical sterilizing agent according to manufacturer's instructions or boiling water for 30 minutes.
   4. Sterilization
      i. Kills **all** microorganisms.
      ii. Required for all nondisposable surgical instruments.
      iii. Requires autoclave or prolonged immersion in chemical sterilizing agent.

E. Recommended immunizations, vaccinations, testing
   1. Regular TB testing
   2. Hepatitis B vaccination series
   3. Tetanus shot
   4. Influenza vaccine
   5. COVID-19 vaccine

Chapter 14

6. MMR vaccine
7. Varicella vaccine
8. Pneumococcal vaccine
9. Pertussis

REVIEW QUESTIONS
(Answers on pg. 420.)

1. Which of the following is an inherited form of chronic anemia, primarily affecting people of African descent?

    A. sickle cell disease

    B. leukemia

    B. hemophilia

    D. multiple myeloma

2. Which of the following are most likely to respond to antibiotic treatment? (Select TWO.)

    A. COVID-19

    B. UTI

    C. influenza

    D. Varicella

    E. strep throat

3. Which of the following is a blood-borne pathogen with substantial risk to healthcare personnel?

    A. hepatitis A

    B. tuberculosis

    C. hepatitis B

    D. RSV

Hematology and Infectious Disease

4. What is the appropriate PPE for a patient with suspected RSV?

    A. self-contained breathing apparatus

    B. gloves only

    C. gloves and face shield

    D. N95 mask

5. Your pediatric patient presents with acute respiratory distress, stridor, and a "barking" cough. You should suspect:

    A. epiglottitis.

    B. RSV.

    C. meningitis.

    D. croup.

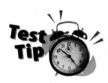

EMT candidates won't get paramedic questions on the certification exam; however, paramedic candidates **will** get EMT questions. Make sure your EMT knowledge is still sharp.

Behavioral Disorders

Chapter 15

I. TERMS TO KNOW

A. **Addiction (drug):** Tolerance and dependence, accompanied by drug-seeking behavior.

B. **Agitated delirium:** Delirium characterized by agitation, aggression, acute distress; aka excited delirium.

C. **Agnosia:** Inability to recognize objects or stimuli (not due to impaired sensory function).

D. **Aphasia:** Loss of ability to express or understand speech.

E. **Apraxia:** Impaired motor activity (not due to impaired sensory function).

F. **Behavioral emergency:** Behavior considered abnormal enough that it requires intervention and alarms the patient or another person.

G. **Delirium:** Acute onset of disorganized thought, often due to correctable causes.

H. **Delusions:** Firmly held beliefs despite being contradicted by what is generally accepted as real or rational.

I. **Dementia:** Slow onset of cognitive deficits. Usually irreversible.

J. **Dependence (drug):** When the body/brain rely on the drug.

K. **Hallucinations:** Sensory perceptions with no basis in reality; often "hearing voices."

L. **Hypochondriasis:** Delusions of serious physical illness.

M. **Paranoia:** Suspicion and mistrust of people or their actions without evidence or justification.

N. **Phobias:** Extreme or irrational fear of something.

O. **Positional asphyxia:** Death due to obstruction of breathing related to body position.

P. **Tolerance (drug):** When an increased dosage is required to achieve the same effects.

Q. **Withdrawal:** Physiological or psychological effects of discontinuing an abused substance.

II. PATHOPHYSIOLOGY OF BEHAVIORAL DISORDERS

A. Biological
   1. Aka "organic" disorder.
   2. Examples: tumors, infection, damage due to drugs or alcohol.
   3. *Note:* Always consider biological causes of unusual behavior, e.g., hypoxia, diabetic emergency, drugs, hypoxia, traumatic brain injury, toxic exposure, etc.

B. Psychosocial
   1. Behavioral abnormalities due to individual personality, unresolved conflicts, coping mechanisms, crisis management, etc.
   2. Psychosocial causes are **not** due to substance abuse or other biological or medical condition.
   3. Examples: anxiety, bipolar disorder, depression, paranoia, phobias, psychosis, schizophrenia.

C. Social
   1. Abnormal behavior due to social situations.
   2. Examples: relationship changes, loss of support system, isolation.

> *Remember:* Do not rush calls involving behavioral patients. They take as long as they take. Utilize locally available resources.

III. MANAGEMENT OF BEHAVIORAL DISORDERS

A. Scene safety actions

  1. Carefully monitor scene for safety.

  2. De-escalate agitated patients.

  3. Have an exit plan.

B. Risk factors for potential violence

  1. Scenes involving alcohol or drug use

  2. Large crowds

  3. Violent incidents (such as domestic disturbances)

  4. Patients who are obviously tense or restless, or have aggressive posture

  5. Patients who are yelling, swearing, or threatening

  6. Suicidal patients

  7. Agitated/excited delirium patients

C. General management of advanced life support patients (Patient Assessment chapter).

D. Listen carefully and ask open-ended questions. Do not interrupt.

E. Do not rush. These scenes often take time.

F. Do not give ultimatums.

G. Be nonjudgmental and honest. Do not threaten or give ultimatums.

H. Maintain safe distance (at eye level when possible). Do not assume threatening posture over patient.

I. De-escalation techniques

  1. Show empathy, be nonjudgmental and honest.

  2. Respect patient's personal space.

  3. Use neutral tone and body language (no yelling).

4. Do not over-react to or ignore challenging questions.
5. Negotiate when possible, but enforce clear boundaries related to safety.
6. Allow silence and time for decision-making.
7. Listen, don't interrupt.
8. Ask open-ended questions.
9. Don't rush patient or issue ultimatums.

IV. MISCELLANEOUS BEHAVIORAL DISORDERS

A. Acute psychosis
   1. Psychosis is a disorder characterized by sudden onset of symptoms including delusions, hallucinations, disorganized speech or behavior, or catatonic behavior.
   2. Symptoms are **not** caused by schizophrenia or bipolar disorder.

B. Delirium
   1. Acute onset (hours to days) of cognitive problems, usually confusion. Other signs and symptoms may include inattention, memory loss, hallucinations.
   2. Often due to treatable medical condition.

C. Dementia
   1. Slow onset (months) of memory impairment and at least one of the following: aphasia, apraxia, agnosia, inability to plan or organize.
   2. Causes include Alzheimer's disease, AIDS, traumatic brain injury, Parkinson's disease.
   3. Unlike delirium, dementia is often irreversible.

D. Schizophrenia
   1. Significant behavioral changes and loss of contact with reality.
   2. Patient often presents with hallucinations, delusions, and depression.

E. Anxiety (panic attack)
   1. Severe apprehension or fear.
   2. Includes panic disorder, phobias, and post-traumatic stress disorder (PTSD).
   3. Signs and symptoms, in addition to extreme fear or anxiety
      i. Palpitations
      ii. Tachypnea
      iii. Diaphoresis
      iv. Trembling
      v. Dyspnea
      vi. Chest pain
      vii. Dizziness

F. Depression
   1. Profound sadness that can be unusually prolonged or severe.
   2. Often accompanied by the following:
      i. Loss of interest in most activities, pleasures.
      ii. Lack of sleep or appetite.
      iii. Lack of concentration.
      iv. Guilt.
      v. Loss of energy.
      vi. Thoughts of suicide.

G. Bipolar disorder
   1. One or more manic episodes (periods of elation), sometimes followed by periods of depression.
   2. Manic episodes may present with:
      i. Inflated self-esteem.
      ii. Highly talkative.
      iii. Decreased sleep.
      iv. Distracted behavior.

Chapter 15

        v. Unrealistic plans.

        vi. Questionable participation in pleasurable activities with consequences, e.g., spending, sexual behavior, business decisions.

H. Somatoform disorders

    1. Physical symptoms with no apparent physiological cause.

    2. Patient may present with the following:

        i. Preoccupation with physical symptoms.

        ii. Unexplained loss of function, e.g., blindness, paralysis.

        iii. Hypochondriasis.

        iv. Perceived defect in physical appearance.

        v. Unexplained pain.

I. Anorexia

    1. Excessive fasting due to intense fear of obesity.

    2. Patients often perceive themselves as overweight when they are not.

J. Bulimia

    1. Recurrent episodes of binge eating followed by self-induced vomiting or diarrhea or excessive dieting or exercise.

    2. Patients are aware that the behavior is abnormal.

K. Suicide

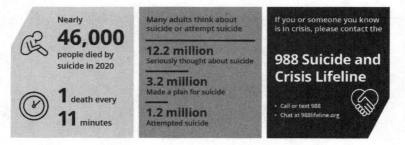

Figure 15-1. Suicide Prevention

National Suicide Prevention Week is September 4th–September 10th and is part of Suicide Prevention Awareness Month. | Hopewell Therapeutic Farm | 440.426.2000 (hopewellcommunity.org)

1. A top 10 leading cause of death for ages 10–64.
2. Second-leading cause of death for ages 10–14.
3. Females are more likely to attempt suicide, while males are more likely to die by suicide.
4. Self-inflicted gunshot wounds and overdose account for more than 75% of suicides.
5. 40% of transgender individuals have attempted suicide.
6. Risk factors
    i. Previous suicide attempts (80% of successful suicide victims have made previous attempts)
    ii. Depression (severely depressed patients 500 times more likely to attempt suicide)
    iii. History of alcohol abuse, drug abuse, child abuse
    iv. Loss of spouse (divorce or death)
    v. Increased isolation, such as living alone
    vi. Loss of loved one, job, money
    vii. Lack of access to mental health services
    viii. Physical or mental stress
    ix. Expresses a clear plan for committing suicide and has the means to carry out suicide attempt

L. Excited delirium, aka agitated delirium
1. Sudden onset of extreme agitation and combative behavior.
2. Causes include drugs (often cocaine) and psychiatric illness.
3. Almost all excited delirium patients present with:
    i. High pain tolerance.
    ii. Tachypnea.
    iii. Diaphoresis.
    iv. Agitation.
    v. Noncompliance toward authorities.
    vi. Do not tire.
    vii. Excessive strength.

4. High risk of sudden cardiac arrest. Physical restraint is a risk factor for sudden cardiac arrest in these patients.
5. Chemical restraint medications may be indicated for patients with a high risk of violence.
6. *Note:* Concurrent use of benzodiazepines and olanzapine is not recommended due to reports of fatalities.

M. Common antidepressant medications
   1. Selective serotonin reuptake inhibitors (SSRIs)
      i. Examples: Prozac, Paxil, Lexapro, Zoloft
   2. Serotonin-norepinephrine reuptake inhibitors (SNRIs)
      i. Example: Cymbalta
   3. Tricyclic antidepressants (TCAs)
      i. Examples: Amitril, Elavil, Tofranil
   4. Monoamine oxidase inhibitors (MAOs)
      i. Examples: Marplan, Nardil, Parnate

N. Special situations
   1. Restraint of violent patients
      i. Follow local protocols regarding medical/legal considerations of patient restraint.
      ii. Leave the scene if weapons are present.
      iii. Only restrain the patient if you have adequate resources immediately available.
      iv. Methods of restraint
         ➤ Verbal de-escalation
         ➤ Chemical restraint
            — Examples: ketamine, benzodiazepines (e.g., midazolam), olanzapine.
         ➤ Physical restraint
            — Have at least 5 people whenever possible (each extremity and the head).
            — Avoid hard restraints when possible.

Behavioral Disorders

- Secure all four extremities.
- Position patient to prevent suffocation, aspiration, or circulatory compromise.
- Continuously monitor patient's airway, breathing, and level of consciousness.
- Always take the patient seriously if they say "I can't breathe."

➤ Never:
- Never secure a patient in the prone position or hog tie.
- Never "sandwich" patient between two backboards.
- Never constrict the patient's neck or compromise the airway.

V. SUBSTANCE ABUSE

A. Pathophysiology of substance abuse

1. People are not equally vulnerable to developing substance-related disorders.
2. Some individuals have lower levels of self-control, which may be physiologically or psychologically based.

B. Signs of substance abuse

1. Taking a substance in larger amounts, or for longer than is recommended or intended.
2. Wanting to stop using a substance, but unable to do so.
3. Spending excessive time acquiring, using, or recovering from substance use.
4. Cravings and urges to use a substance or substances.
5. Failure to meet obligations at home, work, or school because of substance use.
6. Continued use of a substance despite damage to personal relationships.
7. Needing more of a substance to achieve the desired effect.
8. Withdrawal symptoms, which are relieved by continued use of a substance.

C. Drug tolerance, dependence, addiction, withdrawal

1. Tolerance: Occurs when a person requires an increased dosage to maintain the same effects.
2. Dependence: Occurs when body and brain rely on the drug.
3. Addiction: Requires tolerance and dependence and accompanied by compulsive drug-seeking behaviors.
4. Withdrawal: Physiological and/or psychological effects of discontinuing an abused substance.

REVIEW QUESTIONS
(Answers on pg. 420.)

1. Which of the following are known risk factors for potential violence? (Select THREE.)
   A. all patients with mental illness
   B. scenes involving alcohol or drugs
   C. large crowds
   D. unresponsive patients
   E. agitated delirium patients
   F. elderly patients

2. Which of the following is recommended on calls involving behavioral disorders?
   A. transport quickly
   B. provide clear ultimatums
   C. use open-ended questions
   D. use a firm, loud tone

Behavioral Disorders

3. Family states that your elderly patient has had a slow onset of memory impairment over the last year. You should suspect:

    A. delirium.

    B. schizophrenia.

    C. depression.

    D. dementia.

4. Excessive fasting due to intense fear of obesity is known as:

    A. anorexia.

    B. bulimia.

    C. somatoform disorder.

    D. acute social disorder.

5. What is the national Suicide and Crisis Lifeline?

    A. 4-1-1

    B. 1-1-9

    C. 9-8-8

    D. 9-9-9

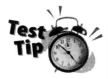

You are at the halfway point of your exam preparation. Keep up the good work! Are you on track to take the certification exam when you planned? Remember, completing your exam prep in under 30 days is highly recommended.

Eye, Ear, Nose, and Throat Disorders

Chapter 16

I. TERMS TO KNOW

A. **Conjunctiva:** Membrane covering the eye and inside of eyelid.

B. **Cornea:** Transparent anterior portion of the eye.

C. **Epiglottitis:** Inflammation of the epiglottis.

D. **Epistaxis:** Nosebleed.

E. **Morgan lens:** Device used to irrigate the eyes. Resembles a contact lens that is connected to tubing.

F. **Sinusitis:** Infection or inflammation of the sinuses.

II. PATHOPHYSIOLOGY OF EYE INJURIES

A. About 27% of serious eye injuries lead to legal blindness.

B. Most common eye injuries

1. Corneal abrasion

2. Foreign objects in eye

3. Chemical burns

4. Blunt trauma

III. CONDITIONS AND INJURIES OF THE EYE

A. Increased ocular pressure

1. An acute increase in ocular pressure is a medical emergency regardless of the cause.

2. Signs and symptoms of increased ocular pressure
    i. Abnormal pupillary response
    ii. Loss of vision or visual acuity
    iii. Halos, blurred vision, tunnel vision, blind spots
    iv. Impaired eye movement
    v. Associated trauma
    vi. Eye pain

B. Eye disease emergencies (all can cause blindness)
   1. Central retinal artery occlusion: Blood supply to retina becomes blocked.
   2. Diabetic retinopathy: Damaged blood vessels in the retina due to diabetes.
   3. Glaucoma: Condition causing increased intraocular pressure.
   4. Macular degeneration: Deterioration of the retina.
   5. Retinal detachment: Separation of retina from supporting structures.

C. Miscellaneous eye conditions
   1. Cataract: Clouding of the lens of the eye.
   2. Conjunctivitis (aka "pink eye"): Infection or inflammation of the conjunctiva.
   3. Corneal abrasion: Painful abrasion to cornea, often caused by direct trauma, foreign body, or contact lenses.
   4. Papilledema: Inflammation of the optic nerve.
   5. Sty or stye: Infection of the eyelid.

D. Contact lenses
   1. Contact lenses do not usually need to be removed unless there are chemical burns to the eyes.
       i. Hard lenses: Remove using specialized suction cup moistened with sterile water.
       ii. Soft lenses: Remove by pinching lens with thumb and index finger.

Eye, Ear, Nose, and Throat Disorders

    E. Impaled objects

        1. Do **not** remove impaled objects from the eye.

        2. Stabilize object and keep both eyes closed.

    F. Blunt trauma

        1. Can cause minor injury (such as a black eye) or more serious injury (such as orbital fracture).

        2. Orbital fracture

            i. Indicates significant trauma; consider possible traumatic brain injury.

            ii. Signs and symptoms: Visual disturbances, double vision, deformity around orbit, inability to move eye in an upward gaze.

    G. Chemical burns

        1. Immediately and continuously irrigate they eyes with sterile saline.

        2. Avoid irrigating chemicals from one eye into the other.

        3. Consider use of Morgan lens to irrigate the eyes per local protocol.

> ➤ *Remember:* An IV bag of 0.9% sodium chloride ("normal saline") connected to blood tubing connected to a nasal cannula allows for continuous irrigation of the eyes. Place patient supine and place the nasal cannula on the bridge of nose to irrigate medial to lateral (no chemical runoff from one eye to the other).

IV. CONDITIONS OF THE EAR

    A. Labyrinthitis: Irritation and swelling of inner ear. Often causes vertigo, loss of balance, dizziness, nausea & vomiting (N&V).

    B. Ménière disease: Similar presentation to labyrinthitis, but can be progressive.

    C. Otitis externa: Aka swimmer's ear. Inflammation or infection of the outer ear.

Chapter 16

    D. Otitis media: Inflammation or infection of the middle ear.

    E. Tympanic rupture: Ruptured eardrum.

V. CONDITIONS OF THE NOSE AND THROAT

    A. Epistaxis (nosebleed)
1. Anterior nosebleeds
   i. Most nosebleeds (90%) are anterior and minor.
   ii. Bleeding is usually through the nares.
2. Posterior nosebleeds
   i. Posterior nosebleeds are usually arterial and can bleed profusely.
   ii. Blood often drains into nasopharynx and mouth.
   iii. Increased risk of swallowing blood and vomiting.
3. Causes of nosebleeds
   i. Low humidity
   ii. Allergies
   iii. Digital trauma
   iv. Miscellaneous drugs and medications
   v. Deviated septum
   vi. Tumors
   vii. Coagulation disorders
   viii. Hypertension
4. Management
   i. Manual pressure (pinching the nose).
   ii. Nasal tampons, per local protocol.
   iii. Consider antiemetics as indicated.
   iv. Patient may need cauterization at appropriate facility.
   v. Rule out hypertension, use of blood thinners, head injury, etc.

B. Epiglottitis: See Hematology and Infectious Disease chapter for additional information.

C. Oral candidiasis
1. Aka "thrush."
2. Fungal infection of the mouth.
3. Most common in infants, diabetics, AIDS patients, and those taking antibiotics.

D. Ludwig's angina
1. Oral inflammation under the tongue.
2. Can develop rapidly and can cause airway obstruction.
3. In severe cases, surgical cricothyrotomy may be needed.

E. Temporomandibular joint syndrome (TMJ)
1. Problem with joint between temporal bone and mandible.

REVIEW QUESTIONS
(Answers on pg. 421.)

1. Inflammation or infection of the conjunctiva is known as:
    A. cataract.
    B. pink eye.
    C. papilledema.
    D. stye.

2. Your patient has an impaled object in the left eye. You should:
    A. remove the object and keep both eyes open.
    B. remove the object and keep the injured eye closed.
    C. stabilize the object and close the injured eye.
    D. stabilize the object and close both eyes.

Chapter 16

3. Which of the following is recommended for patients with epistaxis?
   A. antiemetics
   B. nitroglycerin
   C. tranexamic acid
   D. epinephrine

4. Which of the following can develop rapidly and cause upper airway obstruction?
   A. thrush
   B. TMJ
   C. Ludwig's angina
   D. Ménière disease

5. Your patient has a chemical burn to the eyes. You should:
   A. close and bandage both eyes.
   B. continuously irrigate both eyes.
   C. identify the appropriate antidote.
   D. assess visual acuity in both eyes.

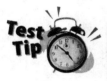

> Expose yourself to as many **good** practice questions as possible (try for at least 100 per NREMT category). Use them to test your knowledge and generate any additional flashcards you might need. Good questions will:
>
> 1. be based on current national guidelines (National Emergency Medical Services Educational Standards, American Heart Association, etc.).
>
> 2. provide a rationale for the correct answer.

Musculoskeletal Disorders

I. TERMS TO KNOW

A. **Lupus:** Chronic autoimmune disease.

B. **Osteoporosis:** Loss of bone density.

C. **Pathological fracture:** Bone fracture caused by disease.

D. **Gout:** A form of inflammatory arthritis.

II. MISCELLANEOUS NONTRAUMATIC MUSCULOSKELETAL CONDITIONS

A. Carpal tunnel syndrome
   1. A repetitive motion condition caused by pressure on the median nerve in the wrist.
   2. Causes numbness, weakness, tingling, or pain anywhere from fingers up to forearm.
   3. A common work-related condition, e.g., keyboarding, tools.

B. Osteoarthritis (OA) (aka degenerative joint disease)
   1. OA is the most common cause of chronic disability in older adults.
   2. Obesity increases the risk of OA.
   3. Causes pain, stiffness, and limited range of motion (usually worse in the morning and improves with movement).

Chapter 17

C. Osteoporosis
   1. Loss of bone density. Most common form of bone disease.
   2. Asymptomatic until late in disease process; then can cause bone pain, tenderness, pathological fracture.

D. Degenerative disk disease
   1. Typically, a normal age-related degeneration of spinal disks.
   2. Common cause of low back pain, especially in elderly.

E. Rheumatoid arthritis
   1. Inflammation and damage to joints and surrounding tissues caused by immune system attacking its own tissue.
   2. Can occur at any age and usually affects wrists, fingers, knees, ankles, feet.
   3. Causes joint swelling, pain, stiffness, and deformity.

F. Ankylosing spondylitis
   1. Inflammatory arthritis typically affecting the spine.
   2. Spine becomes stiff and flexed, causing bent-over walk.
   3. *Note:* Patient's spine may be inflexible. Do **not** attempt to move spine.

G. Lupus
   1. Chronic autoimmune disease affecting skin, joints, kidneys.
   2. Causes chronic inflammation, joint pain, possible fatigue, fever.

H. Gout
   1. A form of inflammatory arthritis caused by uric acid in the joints.
   2. Causes severe pain, swelling, fever.
   3. Can cause severe pain between foot and great toe.

I. Fibromyalgia
   1. Chronic, widespread pain in muscles with tender spots or "trigger points."

2. May be associated with fatigue, anxiety, depression, sleep, or concentration problems.

REVIEW QUESTIONS
(Answers on pg. 421.)

1. Which of the following is an autoimmune disease that causes inflammation and damage to joints and surrounding tissue?

    A. rheumatoid arthritis

    B. osteoporosis

    C. fibromyalgia

    D. carpal tunnel syndrome

2. Your patient complains of fever and severe pain between his foot and great toe. The pain came on suddenly while sleeping. You should suspect:

    A. lupus.

    B. gout.

    C. ankylosing spondylitis.

    D. fibromyalgia.

3. Chronic, widespread pain associated with fatigue, anxiety, or depression is known as:

    A. gout.

    B. lupus.

    C. rheumatoid arthritis.

    D. fibromyalgia.

4. Which of the following is the most common cause of chronic disability in older adults?

    A. degenerative disk disease

    B. osteoarthritis

    C. rheumatoid arthritis

    D. lupus

Chapter 17

5. What is the most common form of bone disease?
   A. osteoporosis
   B. osteoarthritis
   C. ankylosing spondylitis
   D. fibromyalgia

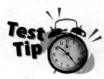

Use practice questions to target your study material. Consider making flashcards.

1. Don't make a flashcard out of a specific practice question you missed. Instead, focus on the content that will help you get any similar question correct next time.

2. Keep your flashcards short and to the point so you have less to memorize.

3. Good practice questions provide a rationale for the correct answer. If you miss a practice question, look at the rationale to see if it can be used to make a flashcard.

4. Missing one practice question can lead to several good flashcards.

PART VI
TRAUMA

Chapter 18

Soft Tissue and Orthopedic Injuries

I. TERMS TO KNOW

- **A. Contusion:** Bruise.

- **B. Crush syndrome:** Systemic complications of a crush injury.

- **C. Dislocation:** Injury where bone is displaced from the joint.

- **D. Displaced fracture:** Fractured ends move from their normal position.

- **E. Hematoma:** Collection of blood beneath the skin.

- **F. Hemostasis:** The body's attempt to control bleeding.

- **G. Nondisplaced fracture:** Bones remain aligned after fracture.

- **H. Occlusive dressing:** Airtight dressing.

- **I. Poikilothermia:** Inability to regulate core body temperature.

- **J. Rhabdomyolysis:** Syndrome due to muscle necrosis and release of toxins into bloodstream.

- **K. Sprain:** Ligament injury.

- **L. Strain:** Muscle or tendon injury.

II. ANATOMY & PHYSIOLOGY REVIEW

Note: See "Integumentary System" in the online Anatomy & Physiology Review at *www.rea.com/paramedic*.

Chapter 18

III. WOUND HISTORY

   A. Time of injury?

   B. Mechanism of injury?

   C. Any other associated injuries?

   D. Signs of shock?

   E. Severity of pain?

   F. Bleeding disorders, diabetes, immunocompromised?

   G. Blood thinners, beta-blockers, etc.?

   H. Tetanus?

   I. Closure (sutures) indicated?

IV. WOUND ASSESSMENT

   A. Deformity, crepitus?

   B. Foreign bodies?

   C. Edema?

   D. Distal pulse, motor, sensation?

V. WOUNDS REQUIRING EMERGENCY CARE

   A. Cosmetic regions

   B. Gaping wounds

   C. Wounds over joints

Soft Tissue and Orthopedic Injuries

   D. Degloving injuries

   E. Ring finger injuries

   F. Continued bleeding

   G. Animal bites

   H. Open fractures

   I. *Note:* Wound infection occurs in up to 50% of human bites.

VI. SOFT TISSUE INJURIES

   A. Closed soft tissue injuries
   1. Contusion
   2. Hematoma
   3. Pressure wound
   4. Crush injury and crush syndrome

   B. Open soft tissue injuries
   1. Abrasions
   2. Lacerations
   3. Avulsions
   4. Amputations
   5. Bites (risk of infection and rabies)
   6. Punctures/impaled objects
   7. Blast injuries
   8. High-pressure injection injuries (characterized by a small puncture wound that can cause extensive tissue damage and potential loss of limb)

   C. Crush injuries
   1. Compression injury that can be open or closed.

2. Increased risk of crush syndrome if an extremity has been trapped for a prolonged period (4+ hours).
3. Crush injury can cause intracellular release of potassium and cause cardiac dysrhythmias.
4. Patients with suspected crush injury should be placed on continuous ECG monitoring.

D. Management of significant closed soft tissue injuries ("RICES")
1. **R:** Rest
2. **I:** Ice
3. **C:** Compression
4. **E:** Elevate
5. **S:** Splint

E. Management of significant open soft tissue injuries
1. General management of soft tissue injuries
    i. Control bleeding.
        ➤ Direct pressure (manual or mechanical as indicated).
        ➤ Tourniquet as indicated for life-threatening extremity bleeding uncontrollable with direct pressure.
    ii. Splinting as indicated to limit motion and reduce bleeding.
    iii. Pain management, such as cold pack (avoid placing directly on injury) and analgesics as indicated and per local protocol.
    iv. Tetanus
        ➤ Remind patient to be sure tetanus immunization is current.
        ➤ Booster at least every 10 years.
2. Risk factors for infection
    i. Wound contamination
    ii. Age
    iii. Illness, e.g., diabetes, chronic obstructive pulmonary disease, cancer, anemia
    iv. Immunosuppressant meds

Soft Tissue and Orthopedic Injuries

- **F.** Special situations
    1. Patients exposed to less lethal weapons (such as a Taser)
        - ➤ Patients exposed to less lethal weapons, such as a Taser or stun gun, should be treated and transported unless **all** of the following criteria are met:
            - Glasgow Coma Scale score of 15.
            - Pulse rate under 110 beats per minute (in adults).
            - Respiratory rate under 12 per minute (in adults).
            - Normal SpO_2.
            - Normal 12-lead ECG.
            - Systolic blood pressure over 100 mmHg (in adults).
            - Dart **not** in eye, face, neck, axilla, groin, or breast (females).
            - No associated injury, illness, or psychiatric condition.
    2. Pressure wounds
        i. Caused by prolonged compression of soft tissue.
            - ➤ Bedridden patients
            - ➤ Falls where patient cannot move for several hours.
            - ➤ Entrapment.
            - ➤ Prolonged immobilization on a spine board
    3. Open neck wound
        i. Apply an occlusive dressing to prevent air embolism.
        ii. Control bleeding without cutting off blood flow or compressing the trachea.
    4. Impaled objects
        i. Do **not** remove impaled objects except in extreme circumstances, e.g., impaled object in cheek and unable to control airway or impaled object that will not allow CPR in a cardiac arrest patient.
        ii. Control bleeding with direct pressure around impaled object.
        iii. Stabilize impaled object in place.

Chapter 18

5. Amputation
    i. Manage patient first and amputated part second.
    ii. Rinse gross contaminants off amputated part.
    iii. Wrap part in saline-soaked sterile dressing.
    iv. Place part in plastic bag and keep cool (do **not** freeze).
    v. Do **not** submerge in water.
    vi. Transport amputated part with patient when possible.

 VIII. ORTHOPEDIC INJURIES

A. Fracture classification and common causes
   1. Linear fracture: Parallel to long axis of bone (low injury stress).
   2. Transverse fracture: Straight across bone (direct blow).
   3. Oblique fracture: An angle across bone (direct or twisting force).
   4. Spiral fracture: Encircles bone (twisting injury).
   5. Impaled fracture: Compression fracture (significant fall).
   6. Pathologic fracture: Atraumatic fracture (disease, cancer, etc.).
   7. Greenstick fracture: Incomplete fracture (occurs in children).
   8. Fatigue fracture: Stress fracture usually in legs or feet (repetitive activities).

B. Dislocations
   1. Subluxation: Partial dislocation of a joint.
   2. Luxation: Complete dislocation.

C. Sprains
   1. Stretching or tearing of ligament, usually due to sudden movement of joint beyond its normal range of motion.
   2. Usually occurs in ankles or knees.
   3. Signs and symptoms include pain, swelling, discoloration.

D. Strains
   1. Muscle or tendon injury due to severe muscle contraction or overstretching.
   2. Signs and symptoms include pain, increased pain on movement, usually only minor swelling.

E. Management of orthopedic injuries
   1. General management of advanced life support (ALS) patients (Patient Assessment chapter).
   2. RICES (rest, ice, compression, elevation, splinting).
      i. Remember to assess distal pulse, motor, sensation before and after splinting.
      ii. Splinting guidelines
         ➤ Splint in normal anatomical position in most cases.
         ➤ Realign angulated long bone fractures per local protocol but **stop** if resistance or severe pain.
         ➤ Do not realign dislocations or fractures close to joint unless distal pulses are absent.
      iii. Ensure bandages and splints are not too tight and compromising distal blood flow.
      iv. *Note:* Orthopedic injuries with absent distal pulses require rapid transport.
   3. Pain management, e.g., cold pack, analgesics.

> ➤ *Remember:* Minimizing pain due to fractures, dislocations, or soft-tissue injuries is an important part of patient care for significant soft-tissue and musculoskeletal injuries.

F. Special situations
   1. Compartment syndrome
      i. Ischemic injury caused by increased pressure and reduced blood flow.
      ii. Often due to crush injury to leg or forearm.

      iii. Signs and symptoms ("The Six Ps")
- Pain
- Pallor
- Paralysis
- Pressure
- Paresthesia
- Pulselessness

      iv. Some patients with compartment syndrome develop poikilothermia (inability to regulate core body temperature).

      v. Management
- This is a limb-threatening injury, especially once extremity is pulseless.
- Immobilize extremity at heart level (not above).
- Isotonic IV fluids may help flush toxins from rhabdomyolysis.

2. Crush syndrome

    i. Caused by prolonged compression force. Ischemic muscle tissue leads to necrosis and rhabdomyolysis.

    ii. Rhabdomyolysis is the rapid destruction of skeletal muscle due to muscle necrosis. Results in release of toxins into the bloodstream that can cause renal failure.

    iii. Management
- General management of ALS patients (Patient Assessment chapter).
  — Ensure high flow oxygen.
  — IV crystalloid fluid bolus (to protect kidneys).
  — Cardiac monitoring (due to risk of hyperkalemia).
  — *Note:* Albuterol small volume nebulizer and IV calcium can reduce risk of hyperkalemia-induced cardiac dysrhythmias.

3. Deep vein thrombosis (DVT)
    i. Signs and symptoms
        ➤ Swelling of extremity
        ➤ Pain in extremity
        ➤ Overly warm extremity
    ii. *Note:* DVT increases the risk of pulmonary embolism (see Pulmonology chapter)
4. Pelvic and femur fractures
    i. 95% of hip fractures are due to fall injuries, usually in females.
    ii. Assess for deformity, swelling, tenderness, instability, crepitus, shortening and rotation of the leg,
    iii. High risk of hemorrhagic shock.
    iv. Treat for shock as indicated.
    v. Consider pelvic binder to reduce bleeding (per local protocol).
    vi. *Note:* Traction splints are indicated for isolated, closed, midshaft femur fractures, but do not delay transport of a high-priority trauma patient to apply a traction splint.
    vii. Rapid transport to appropriate trauma center.

REVIEW QUESTIONS
(Answers on pg. 422.)

1. Which of the following are part of the wound history? (Select THREE.)
    A. time of injury
    B. blood type
    C. previous surgeries
    D. severity of pain
    E. age of patient
    F. last tetanus shot

Chapter 18

2. Where would you assess distal pulses if you suspected an ulnar fracture?

   A. radial pulse
   B. brachial pulse
   C. pedal pulse
   D. ulnar pulse

3. Your patient's arm has been trapped in a stump grinder for almost 4 hours. You should suspect:

   A. angioedema.
   B. crush syndrome.
   C. hypothermia.
   D. gangrene.

4. Your patient was tasered by law enforcement. Which of the following are indications for transport? (Select TWO.)

   A. pulse rate of 120
   B. respiratory rate of 20
   C. systolic blood pressure of 110 mmHg
   D. SpO$_2$ of 98%

5. Your patient has a large open neck wound. You should:

   A. pack the wound.
   B. apply a tourniquet.
   C. apply an occlusive dressing.
   D. place the patient supine.

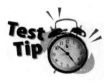

You will see performance scenario questions on the national certification exam. This is a new type of question on the exam. Expect at least two performance scenario questions with 10–12 questions each. To learn more, visit: www.nremt.org/Document/Paramedic-Full-Education-Program-Pathway

Burn Injuries

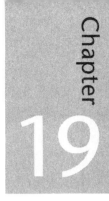

I. TERMS TO KNOW

A. **Body surface area (BSA):** The amount of skin involved in bury injury. Expressed as a percentage of total body surface area.

B. **Circumferential burn:** A burn around the full circumference of an area, e.g., arm, chest, etc.

C. **Eschar:** Leathery, inelastic skin due to full-thickness burn injury.

II. ANATOMY & PHYSIOLOGY REVIEW

Note: See "Integumentary System" in the online Anatomy & Physiology Review chapter at *www.rea.com/paramedic*.

III. PATHOPHYSIOLOGY

A. Most burn injuries occur at home and involve 10% or less of the patient's total body surface area (TBSA).

B. 60% of thermal burns occur in children age 5 or under.

C. 10% of burn injuries require hospitalization.

IV. SYSTEMIC COMPLICATIONS OF SIGNIFICANT BURN INJURIES

A. Infection

B. Hypovolemia

C. Hypothermia

D. Organ failure, such as acute renal failure

E. Respiratory compromise

V. TYPES OF BURN INJURIES

A. Thermal

1. Burn zones

    i. Zone of coagulation: Center of burn and most damaged.

    ii. Zone of stasis: Adjacent to zone of coagulation. Presents with inflammation and decreased perfusion.

    iii. Zone of hyperemia: Farthest from zone of coagulation. Least damaged area of burn.

2. Four phases of injury

    i. Emergent phase

    ➤ Initial response to burn, e.g., pain, anxiety.

    ii. Fluid shift phase

    ➤ Inflammatory response. Causes massive edema in burns over 20% TBSA.

    ➤ Peaks in 6–8 hours, lasts up to 24 hours.

    iii. Hypermetabolic phase

    ➤ Increased metabolic workload and caloric demand due to healing process.

    iv. Resolution phase

    ➤ Rehabilitation phase and development of scar tissue.

v. *Note:* Be alert for burn injuries that may indicate abuse:
   - Explanation inconsistent with injury.
   - Burns to buttocks, between the legs, ankles, wrists, palms, soles.
   - Other suspicious injuries present.
   - Delay in seeking medical attention.

B. Electrical
   1. Damage caused by heat created by body's resistance to flow of electricity.
   2. Damage occurs from the inside out; can result in significant internal damage even with little outward signs of injury.

C. Chemical
   1. Caused by exposure to strong acids or alkalis.
   2. Strong acids can cause coagulation necrosis to skin (limiting depth of burn).
   3. Strong alkalis can cause liquification necrosis, causing much deeper, rapidly penetrating injury.

D. Radiation
   1. Types of radiation
      i. Alpha: Weak. Stopped by skin, clothes, etc.
      ii. Beta: Stronger. Travels several feet. Penetrates clothing, first few layers of skin.
      iii. Gamma: Most powerful. Penetrates body. Stopped by thick concrete or lead.
   2. Protection from radiation injury (the "big three")
      i. Time: Radiation is an accumulative hazard. Limit exposure time and number of exposures.
      ii. Distance: Radiation strength diminishes quickly with distance (exposure at 1 foot distance will be 1/16th that at 4-foot distance).
      iii. Shielding: Get as much shielding as possible between you and source of radiation.

3. Radiation exposure
    i. Below 100 rem: Minimal risk of harm.
    ii. 100–200 rem: Non-life-threatening symptoms.
    iii. 200 rem: Nausea, vomiting, diarrhea within 4 hours.
    iv. 450 rem: Cognitive impairment.
    v. 600 rem: Fatal.
4. Signs and symptoms of radiation sickness
    i. Nausea & vomiting
    ii. Diarrhea
    iii. Weakness
    iv. Confusion

E. Inhalation injury
  1. Burn injuries from enclosed space may cause associated inhalation injury and CO poisoning.
  2. Signs and symptoms of inhalation injury
      i. Confined space mechanism of injury
      ii. Hoarse voice
      iii. Cough
      iv. Dyspnea
      v. Stridor (*Note:* This is a sign of significant partial upper airway obstruction!)
      vi. Singed hair
      vii. Carbonaceous sputum
      viii. Facial burns
      ix. *Note:* Up to 80% of fatal burn injuries involve inhalation injury.

VI. ASSESSMENT OF BURN INJURIES

A. Factors in determining burn severity
  1. Depth of burn
  2. BSA involved

3. Area(s) burned
4. Associated trauma or preexisting conditions
5. Age of patient (under 5 and over 55 at higher risk)

B. Burn depth
1. Superficial, aka first-degree burns
    i. Involves only epidermal layer and possibly upper dermis.
    ii. No blisters!
    iii. Causes pain, redness.
2. Partial, aka second-degree burns
    i. Burns through epidermis and into dermis.
    ii. Causes pain, **blisters**, redness, swelling.
3. Full thickness, aka third-degree burns
    i. Burns through epidermis and dermis into deeper tissue.
    ii. Destroys regenerative/repair process and nerve endings.
    iii. No pain to area of full-thickness burn, but margins can be painful.
    iv. Skin can be white, brown, red, charred, or leathery appearance.
    v. Leads to eschar (inelastic tissue that can compromise blood flow and ventilation with circumferential burns).

C. Total body surface area (TBSA)
1. Rule of nines
    i. Useful for large, contiguous burn areas.
    ii. Do **not** include superficial (first-degree) burns when calculating TBSA.
    iii. See Rule of Nines graphic.
2. Rule of palm
    i. Useful for small, scattered burn injuries.
    ii. The patient's hand (including fingers) = about 1% TBSA.

Chapter 19

D. Special situations
1. Circumferential burns
   i. Full-thickness circumferential burns to an extremity can compromise blood flow due to edema and inelasticity of eschar.
   ii. Circumferential burn to chest can cause respiratory failure due to compromised chest expansion.
2. Abuse
   i. Be alert for signs of abuse with burns involving children and elderly.
   ii. Examples: Circular burns, cigarette burns, stocking pattern burns.
   iii. Report suspected abuse to appropriate authorities.
3. Lightning strikes
   i. Can cause sudden cardiac arrest and respiratory paralysis.
   ii. 70% of survivors experience serious complications.
   iii. One-third of lightning injuries occur indoors! Avoid water and anything plugged in. Stay off concrete floors.
   iv. Do not triage as a normal trauma code due to increased chance of successful resuscitation with rapid defibrillation and ventilatory support.

VII. BURN SEVERITY

A. See table from the American Burn Association. All criteria listed under "Immediate Consultation with Consideration for Transfer" should be considered critical burns.

B. Follow local protocol regarding transport to a burn unit.

VIII. MANAGEMENT OF BURN INJURIES

A. Management of thermal burns
1. Local minor burns over minimal TBSA
   i. Cooling measures, such as cool water.
   ii. Remove constrictive clothing, jewelry.
   iii. Consider pain meds per local protocol.

2. Burns over 10% TBSA
    i. Stop the burning process.
        ➤ If skin is still hot to the touch, apply moist, sterile burn sheet until skin is no longer hot to touch.
        ➤ Quickly replace with dry, sterile burn sheet to reduce risk of hypothermia.

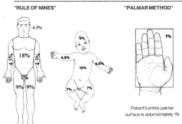

Figure 19-1.
https://ameriburn.org/wp-content/uploads/2023/01/one-page-guidelines-for-burn-patient-referral-16.pdf

ii. Remove clothing, jewelry that may compromise circulation or trap heat.
iii. General management of advanced life support (ALS) patients
iv. Keep warm. Damaged skin has impaired ability to conserve body heat.
v. Apply nonadherent dressings between burns to fingers, toes.
vi. Fluid resuscitation per local protocol.
- Two large-bore IVs with lactated Ringer's (not normal saline).
- Do not place IVs over burned areas.
- Do **not** give a large IV fluid bolus. Utilize Modified Parkland formula per local protocol.
- Modified Parkland formula
  — Indicated for burns over 10% TBSA in children or 20% in adults.
  — 2–4 mL × kg body weight × BSA of burns = IV fluid volume over 24 hours (half administered over first 8 hours).
- Use caution in patients with respiratory compromise due to risk of pulmonary edema.
- Suspect hypovolemia in any burn patient with a heart rate above 140 (100–120 common due to pain or anxiety).
vii. Narcotic analgesia (morphine or fentanyl) IV/IO per local protocol (no IM injections)
viii. Rapid transport to appropriate burn facility (per local protocol)

B. Management of inhalation injury
1. Over 75% of deaths from residential fires involve inhalation injury.
2. Indications for early intubation
   i. Signs of partial airway obstruction, e.g., hoarseness, stridor
   ii. Accessory muscle use, retractions
   iii. Difficulty swallowing
   iv. TBSA over 40%
   v. Deep facial burns

Burn Injuries

   vi. Burns inside mouth
   vii. Inadequate ventilations
   viii. Decreased level of consciousness (LOC)
   ix. Significant edema
   x. Delayed transport
   xi. **Note:** Superficial facial burns, singed hair, and flash burns are **not** indications for early intubation. Administer 100% oxygen and reassess frequently.
3. Management of suspected CO or cyanide poisoning: See Toxicology chapter.
4. Rapid transport to appropriate facility.

C. Management of electrical injury
   1. Heightened scene safety awareness (assume all electrical lines are live).
   2. General management of ALS patients.
   3. Consider spinal precautions.
   4. Anything over 1,000 V is "high voltage."
   5. ECG monitoring due to possible cardiac injury.
   6. *Note:* There can be significant internal damage with little outward signs of injury. Think "iceberg injury"—whatever you can see, there is more that can't be seen.
   7. Rapid transport

D. Management of chemical burns
   1. Heightened scene safety awareness.
   2. Decontaminate patient as indicated.
      i. Brush off dry chemical.
      ii. Remove contaminated clothing.
      iii. Irrigation with large volume of water (in most cases).
      iv. Remove contact lenses if present and irrigate eyes as indicated with continuous water (do not flush chemicals into uninjured eye).
      v. Chemicals requiring special attention (water-reactive)

- ➤ Dry lime: Remove clothing and brush off dry chemical before irrigating with water.
- ➤ Elemental metals: Water on elemental metals (lithium, potassium, sodium, magnesium) produces heat.
        3. General management of ALS patients.
        4. Rapid transport.
    E. Management of radiation injury
        1. Patient should be decontaminated by trained personnel.
        2. *Note:* A decontaminated patient is **not** a source of hazardous radiation.
        3. General management of ALS patients.

IX. SPECIAL SITUATIONS

A. Abuse
    1. Be alert for signs of abuse. Pediatric, elderly, and special needs persons are at higher risk.
    2. Persons who are institutionalized, confused, or unable to communicate are at higher risk.
    3. About 10% of child abuse cases involve burn injuries.
    4. Be alert for "classic dip" or "stocking-pattern" burn pattern to feet, lower legs, buttocks, and genitalia.
        i. No splash marks
        ii. Clear demarcation
        iii. Unexplained or inconsistent explanation

B. Pediatric and elderly patients do **not** tolerate burn injuries well. Hypovolemia and hypothermia can develop rapidly

> ➤ *Remember:* Isolated burn injuries do **not** typically cause the patient to have an altered LOC. If your burn patient has altered mentation, you should suspect other causes (hypoperfusion, head injury, hypoxia, hypoglycemia, inhalation injury, etc.).

REVIEW QUESTIONS
(Answers on pg. 423.)

1. Most thermal burn injuries involve:

    A. abuse.

    B. industrial accidents.

    C. at least 30% TBSA.

    D. children.

2. Which of the following are examples of systemic complications of severe burn injuries? (Select THREE.)

    A. infection

    B. polyuria

    C. hypothermia

    D. respiratory compromise

    E. hydrocephalus

    F. hypertension

3. What is the zone of stasis for a thermal burn?

    A. the center of the burn and the most damaged area

    B. the area farthest from the center of the burn

    C. the area adjacent to the zone of coagulation, that presents with inflammation

    D. the zone with full-thickness destruction and eschar

4. What are the three best ways to protect yourself from radiation injury? (Select THREE.)

    A. Limit exposure time.

    B. Decontaminate frequently.

    C. Take iodine pills within 4 hours of exposure.

    D. Determine the surrounding rem level.

    E. Get as far as possible from source.

    F. Get as much shielding as possible.

Chapter 19

5. Which of the following is recommended for management of critical burn injuries?

   A. Avoid administering narcotic analgesics for pain.
   B. Apply wet, sterile dressings during transport.
   C. Keep the patient cool.
   D. Use lactated Ringer's IV solution for fluid administration.

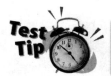

You can take an online, self-paced class on Advanced Burn Life Support (ABLS) through the American Burn Association. For more information, visit: *www.ameriburn.org/education/advanced-burn-life-support-abls/*

Head and Spinal Injuries

Chapter 20

I. TERMS TO KNOW

A. **Anterograde amnesia:** Inability to remember events that occurred after the injury.

B. **Battle's sign:** Bruising to mastoid region (behind ears) indicative of possible basal skull fracture.

C. **Biot's respirations:** Characterized by groups of quick, shallow inspirations, followed by periods of apnea.

D. **Central neurologic hyperventilation:** Deep, rapid respirations (without acetone breath found in Kussmaul respirations).

E. **Cerebral perfusion pressure (CPP):** Mean arterial pressure – intracranial pressure.

F. **Cheyne-Stokes respirations:** Increasing then decreasing tidal volume, followed by period of apnea pressure (intracranial pressure).

G. **Cushing's response (triad):** Hypertension, bradycardia, altered respiratory pattern indicating increased intracranial pressure.

H. **Decerebrate (extensor) posturing:** Posturing with arms extended and toes pointed.

I. **Decorticate (flexor) posturing:** Body extended and arms flexed. Indicates brainstem injury.

J. **Distracting injury:** An injury that produces enough pain to distract the patient from a secondary injury, such as a spinal injury.

K. **Epidural hematoma:** Bleeding between dura mater and skull.

265

Chapter 20

L. **Intracerebral hemorrhage:** Bleeding within the brain.

M. **Intracranial pressure (ICP):** Pressure within the cranium.

N. **Le Fort facial fractures:** Le Fort I: slight instability to maxilla; Le Fort II: fracture of maxilla and nasal bones; Le Fort III: fracture of entire face (zygoma, nasal bone, maxilla).

O. **Priapism:** Persistent penile erection.

P. **Raccoon's eyes:** Bruising around both eyes. Possible indication of orbital fracture or basal skull fracture.

Q. **Retrograde amnesia:** Inability to remember events that occurred before the injury.

R. **Spinal motion restriction:** Technique of minimizing the patient's spine during care and transport. Replaces outdated practice of "full spinal immobilization."

S. **Subdural hematoma:** Bleeding beneath the dura mater, within the meninges (above the brain).

II. ANATOMY & PHYSIOLOGY REVIEW

Note: See "Skeletal System" in the online Anatomy & Physiology Review at *www.rea.com/paramedic*.

III. PATHOPHYSIOLOGY

A. Traumatic brain injury (TBI) accounts for about 30% of all trauma-related deaths.

B. Risk of death doubles for TBI patients with hypotension or hypoxia.

C. Hyperventilation by rescuers contributes to the TBI patient's morbidity and mortality.

> ***Remember:*** Implementation of the Excellence in Prehospital Injury Care (EPIC) TBI guidelines has shown potential positive impact on survival to hospital discharge for patients with severe TBI.
>
> — *JAMA Surgery* 2019;154(7):e191152

IV. TRAUMATIC BRAIN INJURY (TBI)

A. Primary injuries

1. Focal injuries

    i. Cerebral contusion

    ➤ Blunt trauma to brain causing capillary bleeding.

    ➤ Signs and symptoms related to area of brain impacted.

    ➤ *Note:* Patients that deteriorate during prehospital management should be assumed to have something worse than cerebral contusion, e.g., intracranial hemorrhage or increased ICP.

    ii. Intracranial hemorrhage (bleeding within cranium)

    ➤ Epidural hematoma

    — Usually arterial bleeding.

    — Rapid increase in ICP and reduced CPP.

    — Frequently causes loss of consciousness.

    ➤ Subdural hematoma

    — Usually venous bleeding and slow.

    — Patient may be asymptomatic for hours or days.

    — Elderly patients and alcoholics at increased risk.

    ➤ Intracerebral hemorrhage

    — Blood irritates brain tissue.

    — Often rapid onset of progressive stroke-like symptoms.

iii. Cranial fractures
   - Basal skull fractures
     — Commonly associated with facial fractures, cervical spine injury, and intracranial hemorrhage.
     — Signs and symptoms include Battle's sign and raccoon eyes.
   - Facial fractures
     — Le Fort I: Slight instability to maxilla.
     — Le Fort II: Le Fort II: Fracture of maxilla and nasal bones.
     — Le Fort III: Fracture of entire face (zygoma, nasal bone, maxilla).

> *Remember:* Concussion symptoms generally get better over time, not worse. If your patient is getting worse, you should assume a more urgent form of TBI.

2. Diffuse injuries
   i. Concussion
      - Considered a mild diffuse axonal injury.
      - Most common result of blunt head injury.
      - Causes temporary dysfunction without substantial anatomic damage.
      - Signs and symptoms
        — Observable signs
          • Dazed or stunned
          • Confused about events
          • Repeats questions
          • Answers slowly
          • Amnesia about events before or after injury
          • Loss of consciousness
          • Personality changes

- Physical symptoms
  - Headache
  - Nausea & vomiting (N&V)
  - Lack of balance, coordination
  - Fatigued
  - Blurry or double vision
  - Light or noise sensitivity
  - Doesn't "feel right"
- Cognitive symptoms
  - Difficulty concentrating or remembering
  - Feeling slowed down, sluggish, or groggy
- Emotional symptoms
  - Irritable
  - Sad
  - Hyperemotional
  - Nervous

➤ Consider more serious causes if the patient exhibits any of the following:

- Anisocoria
- Unable to awaken patient
- Headache that gets worse
- Repeated vomiting
- Slurred speech or poor coordination
- Seizures
- Difficulty recognizing people or places
- Any signs or symptoms that get worse, not better

ii. Moderate diffuse axonal injury

➤ Caused by shearing, stretching, or tearing of nerve fibers or minor cerebral contusion.

➤ More serious than mild concussion and can result in neurological impairment.

- May be associated with basal skull fracture.
- Signs and symptoms
  - Immediate loss of consciousness followed by confusion
  - Retrograde and anterograde amnesia
  - Headache
  - Neurological deficits
  - Anxiety, mood swings

> *Remember:* You **must** know Cushing's response and what it indicates before taking the certification exam or managing TBI patients as a paramedic.

  iii. Severe diffuse axonal injury
  - Significant disruption of both cerebral hemispheres and brainstem.
  - Often fatal or results in permanent neurological impairment.
  - Presents as unconscious and with signs of increased ICP (Cushing's response).

B. Secondary brain injury
  i. Damage due to factors occurring after primary injury.
  ii. Can be more damaging than the primary injury.
  iii. *Note:* Prehospital management can't reverse primary brain injury, but may be able to reduce secondary injury by:
  - Preventing hypoxia
    - Administration of high-concentration oxygen and monitoring SpO_2 levels.
  - Preventing hypotension
    - Control hemorrhage, management of shock, IV fluid resuscitation.
  - Maintain normal CO_2 levels
    - Continuous capnography.
    - Avoid hyperventilation.

C. General signs and symptoms of brain injury
   i. Altered level of consciousness (LOC)
   ii. Personality changes
   iii. Amnesia
   iv. Cushing's response, aka Cushing's triad (hypertension, bradycardia, altered respirations)
   v. Nausea & vomiting (N&V)
   vi. Pupillary changes
   vii. Posturing (decorticate or decerebrate)
   viii. *Note:* Pediatric patients may present with bulging fontanelles due to increased ICP.

V. SPINAL CORD INJURY

A. Spinal concussion
   1. Temporary and transient disruption of cord function.
   2. No structural damage or permanent deficits.

B. Spinal contusion
   1. Bruising of spinal cord with some tissue damage and edema.
   2. Usually no permanent deficits but longer recovery period than spinal concussion.

C. Spinal compression
   1. Causes include displacement of vertebral body, herniated disk, vertebral bone fragment, or swelling.
   2. Can directly damage spinal cord due to reduced perfusion and ischemia.

D. Cord laceration
   1. Can be caused by bone fragments or other sharp objects driven into cord.
   2. Leads to cord hemorrhage and edema.
   3. Typically causes permanent neurological deficits.

Chapter 20

E. Cord hemorrhage
   1. Can be caused by contusion, laceration, or stretching of cord.
   2. Disrupted blood flow and edema lead to ischemic injury.

F. Cord transection
   1. Partial or complete severing of cord.
   2. Can cause paraplegia, quadriplegia, incontinence, respiratory paralysis.

G. General signs and symptoms of spinal injury
   1. Paralysis
   2. Pain or tenderness along spine
   3. Respiratory impairment
   4. Priapism
   5. Posturing (decorticate or decerebrate)
   6. Incontinence

H. Cord syndromes
   1. Anterior cord syndrome
      i. Usually due to flexion or extension injury.
      ii. Often permanent loss of motor function and pain sensation.
   2. Central cord syndrome
      i. Usually due to hyperextension of cervical spine.
      ii. May be associated with preexisting degenerative disease.
      iii. Causes motor weakness, usually upper extremities and bladder incontinence.
   3. Brown-Sequard syndrome
      i. Usually caused by penetrating injury affecting one side.
      ii. Causes ipsilateral (same side) sensory and motor loss with contralateral (opposite side) loss of pain and temperature perception.
   4. Cauda equina syndrome
      i. Caused by compression of nerve roots at lower end of spine.
      ii. May be caused by herniated disk, tumors, infection.

iii. Can cause pain, bladder and bowel incontinence, lower extremity weakness.

I. Spinal shock

1. Temporary insult to cord. Does not usually cause permanent damage.
2. Causes sensory and motor dysfunction below level of injury.
3. May also cause incontinence, priapism.
4. Causes hypotension due to peripheral vasodilation.

J. Neurogenic shock

1. Caused by disruption of CNS control of autonomic function.
2. Causes widespread vasodilation, relative hypovolemia.
3. Signs and symptoms: See Bleeding and Shock chapter.

> *Remember:* The long spine board is now considered an extrication device. The patient should be removed from the long spine board as soon as possible. Review the NREMT Resource Document on Spinal Motion Restriction/Immobilization prior to taking the national certification exam: *https://www.nremt.org/News/National-Registry-of-EMT-s-Resource-Document-on-Sp*

VI. MANAGEMENT OF HEAD AND SPINAL INJURIES

A. Spinal motion restriction (SMR)

1. The National Association of EMS Physicians, the American College of Emergency Physicians, the American College of Surgeons Committee on Trauma, and the National Registry of EMTs have all issued position statements calling for "spinal motion restriction" to replace "full spinal immobilization." This, in most cases, eliminated the use of the long spine board for immobilization in EMS.
2. Determine need for spinal motion restriction per local protocol.
3. Hazards of full spinal immobilization
    i. True spinal immobilization is almost impossible.
    ii. Increased pain.

iii. Respiratory compromise.

iv. Tissue damage.

v. Some cervical collars may increase ICP.

vi. Delayed transport of high-priority patients.

4. Indications for spinal motion restriction

   i. Blunt trauma with altered LOC.

   ii. Spinal pain or tenderness.

   iii. Neurological compromise, e.g., numbness, tingling, weakness, paralysis.

   iv. Anatomical deformity of the spine.

   v. High-energy mechanisms associated with intoxication, inability to communicate, or distracting injury.

5. Spinal motion restriction procedures

   i. Apply a rigid cervical collar.

   ii. Place patient on stretcher.

   iii. Secure patient using stretcher seat belts.

   iv. SMR does **not** include use of a long spine board.

B. General management of advanced life support patients (Patient Assessment chapter).

C. Determine Glasgow Coma Score (GCS)

1. Adult and pediatric GCS: See Neurology chapter.

D. For TBI patients, special emphasis on:

1. Preventing hypoxia

   i. Administration of high-concentration oxygen and monitoring SpO_2 levels.

   ii. A single episode of hypoxia (SpO_2 below 90%) drastically increases risk of death.

2. Preventing hypotension

   i. Control hemorrhage, management of shock, IV fluid resuscitation.

Head and Spinal Injuries

  ii. A single episode of hypotension (systolic blood pressure below 90 mmHg) drastically increases risk of death.

 3. Maintain normal CO_2 levels

  i. Continuous capnography.

  ii. Avoid hyperventilation during bag-valve-mask (BVM) ventilation.

 4. Manage hypoglycemia

  i. Administer dextrose and thiamine to hypoglycemic patients with suspected TBI per local protocol.

E. Rapid transport to appropriate facility.

VII. SPECIAL SITUATIONS

A. Pediatric patients

 1. Pediatric head injury patients with significant mechanism of injury (MOI) or those who develop symptoms within 72 hours of injury should be transported for evaluation.

 2. Pediatric patients with minor MOI, no loss of consciousness, GCS of 15, and no signs or symptoms of head trauma (other than abrasions) do not typically require transport.

 3. Abuse should be considered for all pediatric patients with head injury.

B. Helmets

 1. In most cases, helmets can be left in place during care and transport as long as the patient can be adequately assessed and managed.

 2. If unable to adequately assess or manage the patient, remove the helmet with minimal movement of the cervical spine.

> ➤ *Remember:* Three critical management principles for a patient with traumatic brain injury are:
>
> 1. No hypotension!
> 2. No hypoxia!
> 3. No hyperventilation!

Chapter 20

REVIEW QUESTIONS
(Answers on pg. 423.)

1. Cushing's triad includes (select THREE):
   A. hypotension.
   B. hypertension.
   C. jugular vein distention.
   D. abnormal respiratory pattern.
   E. tachycardia.
   F. bradycardia.

2. Which of the following is the largest part of the brain, and performs higher cognitive functions?
   A. cerebellum
   B. cerebrum
   C. brainstem
   D. diencephalon

3. Which of the following is true regarding epidural hematomas?
   A. Epidural hematomas often cause a rapid increase in ICP.
   B. Epidural hematomas often cause a rapid increase in CPP.
   C. Epidural hematomas are usually slow venous bleeds.
   D. Epidural hematoma patients are usually asymptomatic for hours to days.

4. Your patient presents with anisocoria. You should suspect:
   A. narcotic overdose.
   B. hypovolemia.
   C. increased ICP.
   D. concussion.

5. Management of a significant TBI patient must include (select THREE):
   A. allowing permissive hypotension.
   B. avoiding hypoxia.
   C. limiting supplemental oxygen administration.
   D. avoiding hypotension.
   E. preventing hyperventilation with the BVM.
   F. reassessing the GCS every 5 minutes.

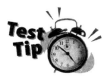

Test Tip: The certification exam is pass/fail. The goal is to demonstrate "entry-level competency." The adaptive technology driving the test is very accurate at assessing competency. If you are prepared, and control your nerves, you will pass!

Chapter 21

Chest, Abdomen, and Pelvic Injuries

I. TERMS TO KNOW

A. **Cullen's sign:** Periumbilical bruising. May indicate internal bleeding, ruptured ectopic pregnancy, acute pancreatitis.

B. **Evisceration:** Open abdominal wound with protruding organs.

C. **Flail chest:** Segment of thorax moves independently due to three or more adjacent ribs fracturing in at least two places.

D. **Grey Turner's sign:** Bruising of the flanks, indicating possible retroperitoneal bleeding, ruptured ectopic pregnancy, or acute pancreatitis.

E. **Hematemesis:** Vomiting blood.

F. **Hematuria:** Blood in urine.

G. **Hemoptysis:** Coughing up blood.

H. **Hemothorax:** Accumulation of blood within pleural space.

I. **Open pneumothorax:** Large, penetrating thoracic trauma that allows air to enter pleural space.

J. **Pelvic binder:** Device used to compress the pelvis with a suspected fracture to minimize internal hemorrhage.

K. **Pericardial tamponade:** Accumulation of fluid in pericardial sac that compromises cardiac filling; aka cardiac tamponade.

L. **Peritoneum:** Tissue covering abdominal cavity, small bowel, and internal organs.

Chapter 21

    M. **Peritonitis:** Inflammation of the peritoneum.

    N. **Pulmonary contusion:** Bruise to lung tissue.

    O. **Pulse pressure:** Systolic pressure − diastolic pressure = pule pressure. Normal pulse pressure is between 40 and 60 mmHg.

    P. **Pulsus paradoxus:** Drop in systolic pressure of at least 10 mmHg during inspiration.

    Q. **Simple pneumothorax:** Closed pulmonary injury where air leaks into pleural space.

    R. **Tension pneumothorax:** Pneumothorax causing progressive build-up of air within pleural space.

    S. **Traumatic asphyxia:** Severe compression of the chest that compromises blood flow.

ANATOMY & PHYSIOLOGY REVIEW/PATHOPHYSIOLOGY

> **Note:** See "Abdominal Cavity" in the online Anatomy & Physiology Review at *www.rea.com/paramedic*.

PATHOPHYSIOLOGY

    A. Chest injuries are the second most common type of nonintentional trauma.

    B. Motor vehicle accidents are the most common cause of chest trauma.

    C. High mortality rates from chest trauma (as high as 60%).

THORACIC TRAUMA

    A. Chest wall injuries

        1. General signs and symptoms of chest wall injuries

            i. Mechanism: blunt or penetrating thoracic trauma

            ii. Pain, crepitus

- iii. Dyspnea (often increasing on inspiration)
- iv. Bruising
- v. Abnormal breath sounds
- vi. Paradoxical motion
- vii. Signs of hypoxia, e.g., low SpO_2

2. Chest wall contusion
   - i. Most common blunt thoracic injury.
   - ii. *Note:* Pediatric patients have chest wall contusion and internal injuries without rib fractures.

3. Rib fractures
   - i. Occur in half of patients with significant thoracic trauma (usually ribs 4 through 8).
   - ii. *Note:* Fractures to ribs 1–3 and 9–12 indicate high likelihood of significant internal injuries.
   - iii. Management
     - ➤ Assess for associated internal injuries.
     - ➤ General management of advanced life support (ALS) patients (Patient Assessment chapter).
     - ➤ Consider analgesics (**not** nitrous oxide).

> ➤ *Remember:* Patients with a suspected flail chest and inadequate breathing **must be ventilated** with a bag-valve-mask (BVM). Bulky dressings, tape, etc., are NOT the appropriate intervention for patients with inadequate ventilation.

4. Flail chest
   - i. Indicates likely associated pulmonary contusion.
   - ii. Can simultaneously reduce respiratory efficiency while increasing respiratory effort.
   - iii. Management
     - ➤ Place patient on injured side if possible, or apply bulky dressing to injured side to help stabilize flail segment.
     - ➤ General management of ALS patients (Patient Assessment chapter).

➤ *Note:* The most important intervention for a suspected flail chest injury with inadequate ventilation is BVM ventilation (**not** a bulky dressing).

B. Pulmonary injuries
   1. Simple pneumothorax (aka closed pneumothorax)
      i. Caused by blunt or penetrating trauma leading to alveolar collapse.
      ii. *Note:* With simple pneumothorax due to penetrating trauma, air enters pleural space through injured airway structures, not directly through penetrating wound.
      iii. Signs and symptoms
         ➤ Mechanism: Thoracic trauma (blunt or penetrating, anterior, posterior, or lateral)
         ➤ Pain, especially on inspiration
         ➤ Dyspnea
         ➤ Tachypnea
         ➤ Subcutaneous emphysema
         ➤ Diminished breath sounds on affected side
         ➤ Signs of hypoxia, e.g., low SpO_2
      iv. Management
         ➤ General management of ALS patients (Patient Assessment chapter).
         ➤ Ensure high-concentration oxygen administration.
   2. Open pneumothorax (aka "sucking chest wound")
      i. Large, penetrating thoracic trauma causes air to enter pleural space directly through the injury during inspiration.
      ii. Signs and symptoms
         ➤ Penetrating thoracic trauma
         ➤ Sucking chest wound, e.g., bubbling air, frothy blood
         ➤ Dyspnea
         ➤ Diminished or absent lung sounds
         ➤ Possible signs of hypovolemic shock

iii. Management

- Apply a ventilated occlusive dressing (upon exhalation).
- General management of ALS patients (Patient Assessment chapter).
- Ensure high-concentration oxygen and initiate BVM ventilation as indicated.
- If condition deteriorates, manually ventilate the occlusive dressing if necessary. If no improvement, assess for tension pneumothorax.
- *Note:* For management of impaled objects, see Soft Tissue and Orthopedic Injuries chapter.

> *Remember:* Narrowing pulse pressure occurs when diastolic pressure rises and systolic pressure falls. Common causes include cardiac tamponade, tension pneumothorax, cardiogenic shock, severe hypovolemia.

3. Tension pneumothorax
   i. Pneumothorax that causes sustained pressure within the thorax.
   ii. Can be caused by simple or open pneumothorax, or positive pressure ventilation.
   iii. Signs and symptoms of tension pneumothorax
   - Thoracic trauma
   - Severe dyspnea
   - Signs of hypoxia, e.g., low SpO_2
   - Progressively diminished to absent lung sounds
   - JVD
   - Hypotension
   - *Note:* Tracheal deviation is a **late** sign and should not be used as an early indicator of tension pneumothorax.
   iv. Management
   - General management of ALS patients (Patient Assessment chapter).

- Decompress affected side as indicated, e.g., needle decompression, as indicated and per local protocol.
4. Hemothorax
    i. Significant hemothorax has a high mortality rate, primarily due to hypovolemic shock.
    ii. Often accompanies pneumothorax, called hemopneumothorax.
    iii. Signs and symptoms
        - Thoracic trauma
        - Signs and symptoms of hypovolemic shock
        - Dyspnea
        - Signs of hypoxia, e.g., low SpO_2
    iv. Management
        - General management of ALS patients (Patient Assessment chapter).
        - BVM ventilations as indicated; consider positive end-expiratory pressure or continuous positive airway pressure.
        - Treat for shock as indicated.
            — IV fluids as indicated.
            — Monitor for pulmonary edema.
5. Pulmonary contusion
    i. Frequently caused by deceleration injury (moving body striking fixed object), or pressure wave caused by high-velocity projectile or explosion.
    ii. Signs and symptoms
        - Thoracic trauma
        - Signs and symptoms of shock
            — Dyspnea
            — Abnormal lung sounds
            — Hemoptysis
            — Signs of hypoxia, e.g., low SpO_2

iii. Management
- ➤ Assess for additional internal injuries.
- ➤ General management of ALS patients (Patient Assessment chapter).

C. Cardiovascular injuries

1. Commotio cordis
   i. Sudden ventricular fibrillation due to blunt chest trauma, e.g., a baseball.
   ii. A leading cause of sudden death in young athletes.
   iii. Prompt recognition, CPR, and defibrillation are essential for survival.
2. Pericardial tamponade
   i. Compromised cardiac filling due to accumulation of blood or other fluid in pericardial sac; aka cardiac tamponade.
   ii. Rare and usually due to penetrating thoracic trauma.
   iii. Signs and symptoms
      - ➤ Beck's triad
        — JVD
        — Narrowing pulse pressure
        — Muffled heart tones
      - ➤ Dyspnea
      - ➤ Signs and symptoms of shock
      - ➤ Pulsus paradoxus
   iv. Management
      - ➤ General management of ALS patients (Patient Assessment chapter).
      - ➤ Aggressive IV fluids to improve cardiac output.
      - ➤ Rapid transport for pericardiocentesis.
3. Traumatic aortic dissection
   i. Almost always fatal within 1 week of injury and usually due to blunt thoracic trauma.

ii. Signs and symptoms

➤ Mechanism: High fall or severe motor vehicle collision

➤ Significant hypotension

➤ Rapid-onset cardiac arrest

➤ Tearing chest or back pain

➤ Pulse deficit between left and right extremities

iii. Management

➤ General management of ALS patients (Patient Assessment chapter).

➤ Conservative IV fluids (mild hypotension may be beneficial).

4. Traumatic asphyxia

i. Severe compression of the chest that compromises blood flow (usually a primary cardiovascular problem, not respiratory).

ii. Signs and symptoms

➤ Mechanism: Significant compression of the chest

➤ Hypotension

➤ Signs and symptoms of shock

➤ Signs of hypoxia, e.g., low SpO_2

➤ Head and neck discoloration

iii. Management

➤ General management of ALS patients (Patient Assessment chapter).

➤ Prepare for BVM ventilation, IV fluid administration, and cardiac dysrhythmias.

V. ABDOMINAL AND PELVIC INJURIES

A. Usually due to motor vehicle collisions with rapid deceleration, crush injury, or compression forces.

B. Trauma is the most common cause of death in pregnant women, often due to abdominal trauma.

C. General signs and symptoms of abdomen and pelvic injury
   1. Mechanism: Blunt or penetrating trauma, often due to motor vehicle collision
   2. Abdominal or flank pain
   3. Referred right shoulder pain
   4. Nausea & vomiting (N&V)
   5. Hematemesis
   6. Hematuria
   7. Rebound tenderness
   8. Guarding (contraction of anterior abdominal muscle)
   9. Abdominal rigidity or distention
   10. Cullen's sign
   11. Grey Turner's sign
   12. Signs and symptoms of shock

D. General management of abdomen and pelvic trauma
   1. General management of ALS patients (Patient Assessment chapter).
   2. Application of a pelvic binder.
      i. Indicated for mechanically unstable pelvic fractures, per local protocol.
      ii. Contraindications include open pelvic fractures, perineal lacerations, obesity, burns.
   3. Treat for shock as indicated.
   4. Rapid transport to appropriate facility.

E. Abdominal evisceration
   1. Bowel is most likely organ to protrude through evisceration opening.
   2. Risk of bowel necrosis due to strangulation or drying.
   3. Management
      i. General management of ALS patients (Patient Assessment chapter).

Chapter 21

      ii. Cover evisceration with moist sterile dressing.

      iii. Cover dressing with occlusive dressing.

  F. Pelvic fracture: See Soft Tissue and Orthopedic Injuries chapter

VI. SPECIAL PATIENTS

A. Pediatric patients
1. Higher risk of being involved in car vs. pedestrian or car vs. bicycle accidents.
2. Chest and abdomen are not well protected.
3. The absence of rib fractures does **not** rule out significant thoracic trauma.

B. Elderly patients
1. Falls are the most common mechanism of injury for elderly patients.
2. Aortic, liver, and spleen injuries more likely.

C. Kidney trauma
1. Patients with kidney trauma are at high risk for other associated trauma.
2. Signs and symptoms of kidney trauma
     i. Flank injuries, pain
     ii. Fractures of lower ribs or lumbar trauma
     iii. Hematuria

REVIEW QUESTIONS
(Answers on pg. 424.)

1. Your trauma patient presents with Grey Turner's sign. You should suspect:
   A. appendicitis.
   B. lower gastrointestinal bleeding.
   C. retroperitoneal bleeding.
   D. acute peritonitis.

2. Your trauma patient presents with abnormal JVD. You should suspect:
   A. simple pneumothorax.
   B. massive hemothorax.
   C. tension pneumothorax.
   D. myocardial contusion.

3. Which of the following indicates a high likelihood of significant internal injuries?
   A. fractures to ribs 1–3
   B. fractures to ribs 4–8
   C. tenderness to palpation of the thorax
   D. increase in pain with deep inspiration

4. Your trauma patient presents with paradoxical motion and hypoxia. You should immediately:
   A. apply a bulky dressing.
   B. apply tape from sternum to spine.
   C. initiate bag-valve-mask ventilation.
   D. determine the $ETCO_2$ level.

Chapter 21

5. Trauma patients with a tension pneumothorax will typically present with severe dyspnea, diminished or absent lung sounds on the affected side, and:

   A. hemodynamic compromise.

   B. normal SpO$_2$ reading.

   C. flat neck veins.

   D. tracheal deviation.

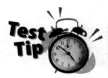

> Expect "priority-of-treatment" questions on the exam. These questions often ask what you should do "first" or "next." Being thoroughly familiar with the patient assessment process will help with these questions. Actions that come earlier in the assessment process (e.g., primary assessment actions) are generally more important than what comes later (secondary assessment actions).

Environmental Emergencies

Chapter 22

I. TERMS TO KNOW

A. **Antivenin:** An antiserum (aka antivenom) containing antibodies against specific poisons, especially those in the venom of spiders, snakes, and scorpions.

B. **Barotrauma:** Injury caused by changes in pressure.

C. **Surfactant:** Alveolar substance that keeps alveoli open.

D. **Tinnitus:** Ringing in the ears.

II. PATHOPHYSIOLOGY OF HEAT AND COLD DISORDERS

A. Heat generation

   1. Increased activity
   2. Increased metabolism
   3. Shivering

B. Heat loss

   1. Conduction: Direct contact with colder object.
   2. Convection: Heat loss to air currents.
   3. Radiation: Body's normal method of dispersing heat to the environment.
   4. Evaporation: Evaporation of water or sweat.
   5. Respiration: Loss of warm, humidified air during exhalation.

C. Predisposing factors for heat and cold emergencies
   1. Age (pediatrics and geriatrics at increased risk)
   2. Health (chronically ill patients at increased risk)
   3. Medications (many meds interfere with defense mechanisms)
D. Physiological response to heat and cold
   1. Cold: Typically causes peripheral vasoconstriction and slowing metabolic rate, e.g., pale, cool skin; decreased pulse rate.
   2. Heat: Typically causes peripheral vasodilation and increasing metabolic rate, e.g., flushed skin, increased pulse rate.

III. HEAT DISORDERS

A. General signs and symptoms
   1. Diaphoresis
   2. Warm, flushed skin
   3. Increased metabolic state

B. Heat cramps
   1. Non-life-threatening.
   2. Caused by exertion, dehydration, possible electrolyte imbalance.
   3. Signs and symptoms
      i. Cramps in arms, legs, sometimes abdomen
      ii. Dizzy, weak
      iii. Warm, wet skin
      iv. *Note:* Patients will be alert, probably with elevated but stable vitals.
   4. Management
      i. Remove patient from hot environment and cease exertional activities.
      ii. Oral rehydration if patient alert with stable airway and no nausea & vomiting (N&V).
      iii. Intravenous (IV) fluids as indicated.
      iv. *Note:* Never administer salt tablets.

Environmental Emergencies

C. Heat exhaustion
1. Mild to moderate systemic heat emergency caused by dehydration and electrolyte loss.
2. Can progress to heat stroke if not managed.
3. Signs and symptoms
    i. Passive or active exposure to hot environment, e.g., home without air conditioning or working outside
    ii. Cool, diaphoretic skin
    iii. Increased metabolic activity, e.g., tachypnea, tachycardia
    iv. Weakness
    v. N&V
    vi. Possible muscle cramps
    vii. *Note:* If patient presents with central nervous system compromise, e.g., altered level of consciousness (LOC), treat for heat stroke immediately.
4. Management
    i. General management of advanced life support (ALS) patients (Patient Assessment chapter) with emphasis on:
        ➤ Remove from hot environment.
        ➤ Begin cooling measures (**not** to point of shivering).
        ➤ Oral or IV fluid rehydration as indicated.
        ➤ Treat for hypovolemic shock as indicated.
    ii. Monitor for signs of impending heat stroke.

> ➤ *Remember:* Wet skin does **not** rule out heat stroke. During heat stroke, the patient will stop sweating. In a hot, dry environment this will lead to hot, dry skin; however, in a humid environment, the skin can stay wet even without active sweating.

D. Heat stroke
1. The most life-threatening systemic heat emergency.
2. Uncontrolled hyperthermia due to loss of temperature regulation ability.
3. Risk of acute, irreversible damage to vital organs.

4. Can be exertional or nonexertional.
5. Signs and symptoms
   i. Altered or decreased LOC
   ii. Usually hot/dry skin due to loss of sweat mechanism (*Note:* Patient may still be diaphoretic in high-humidity environment.)
   iii. Core temp usually greater than 104°F (40.6°C)
   iv. Abnormal respirations
   v. Signs of shock, e.g., tachycardia, hypotension
   vi. Seizures
6. Management
   i. **Must** remove patient from hot environment.
   ii. Initiate rapid cooling measures (target: 102°F/39°C).
      ➤ Perform en route to hospital.
      ➤ Remove clothing, cover with sheets soaked in tepid water.
   iii. General management of ALS patients with emphasis on:
      ➤ Treating for shock.
      ➤ ECG monitoring for dysrhythmias.
   iv. Rapid transport.

IV. COLD DISORDERS

A. Frostbite
   1. Superficial frostbite (aka frostnip) causes redness, blanching, and loss of sensation. Little risk of permanent injury.
   2. Deep frostbite
      i. Affects deep tissue layers.
      ii. White, hard appearance to skin with loss of sensation.
      iii. Management
         ➤ Remove from cold environment.
         ➤ Assess for possible hypothermia.

- Do not allow tissue to refreeze.
- Do **not** massage frozen tissue.
- Apply dry, sterile dressing and elevate.
- Transport for rewarming.
- Consider analgesic meds as indicated and per local protocol.

3. Trench foot
   i. Aka immersion foot.
   ii. Similar to frostbite; occurs when tissue immersed in cold water for prolonged period.
   iii. Management includes drying, warming, and elevating feet.

> *Remember:* Assessing mentation and LOC can be done much faster than obtaining a core temperature. Patients with an altered or decreased LOC are always a high priority. Do not delay transport of a high-priority patient to obtain a core temperature.

B. Hypothermia
   1. Potentially life-threatening systemic cold emergency.
   2. Core temp below 95°F (35°C).
      i. Mild hypothermia: Core temp 90–95°F (32°C) with signs and symptoms.
      ii. Moderate hypothermia: Core temp 82–90°F (28–32°C)
      iii. Severe hypothermia: Core temp below 82°F (28°C) with signs and symptoms.
   3. Signs and symptoms
      i. Altered LOC (mild)/unresponsive (severe)
      ii. Tachycardia (mild)/bradycardia (severe)
      iii. Tachypnea (mild)/bradypnea (severe)
      iv. Shivering (mild)/loss of shivering (severe)
      v. Atrial fibrillation (most common hypothermic dysrhythmia)
      vi. Coma, apnea, ventricular fibrillation, asystole (severe)

4. Management
    i. Remove from cold environment.
    ii. Remove wet clothes.
    iii. Passive rewarming measures, e.g., blankets.
    iv. Avoid rough handling (can induce ventricular fibrillation [VF]).
    v. Monitor core temperature.
    vi. ECG monitoring.
    vii. Prolong pulse check due to chance of severe bradycardia.
        ➤ Patients with a pulse
            — General management of ALS patients (Patient Assessment chapter).
            — Rapid transport.
        ➤ Cardiac arrest patients
            — Begin CPR.
            — Advanced Cardiovascular Life Support (ACLS) guidelines based on core temp.
                • Core temp below 86°F (30°C):
                    – If VF, defibrillate **once** at 360 J or biphasic equivalent.
                    – Continue CPR.
                    – No medications or further defibrillation.
                • Core temp above 86°F (30°C):
                    – Continue CPR.
                    – Defibrillate and administer meds per standard ACLS guidelines.
    viii. Contraindications for initiating resuscitation of hypothermic patient
        ➤ Submersion greater than 1 hour.
        ➤ Core temp below 50°F (10°C).
        ➤ Obvious fatal injuries.
        ➤ Chest wall rigidity prevents CPR.

ix. *Note:* Do **not** discontinue resuscitation of patient that is still hypothermic ("patients are not dead until they are warm and dead").

V. DROWNING

A. Pathophysiology of drowning incident
   1. Victim (at least the airway) enters water
   2. Breath holding
   3. Water swallowing
   4. Laryngospasm
   5. Hypoxia
   6. Airway relaxes
   7. Water enters lungs
   8. Surfactant washout
   9. Cardiac arrest

B. Mammalian diving reflex: Exposure to near-freezing water can rapidly slow metabolic rate and improve survival rates.

C. Management of drowning incident
   1. Remove patient from water only if safe to do so. Initiate spinal precautions as indicated.
   2. Avoid placing patient on surface that can cause surface burns, e.g., hot concrete.
   3. Aggressive management of ABCs (Airway, Breathing, Circulation) as quickly as possible, while still in water if possible. Prepare for vomiting.
   4. CPR and defibrillation as indicated
   5. **Remember:** Initiate CPR for unresponsive pediatric patient with a pulse below 60 beats per minute.
   6. Manage hypothermia as indicated (wet patients lose body heat rapidly).

DIVING EMERGENCIES

A. Gas laws
   1. Boyle's law: Volume of a gas is inversely proportional to its pressure.
   2. Dalton's law: Total pressure of mixed gases is equal to sum of partial pressures of each gas.
   3. Henry's law: Amount of gas dissolved in a given volume of fluid is proportional to the pressure of the gases above it.

B. Diving emergencies
   1. Descent barotrauma, aka "the squeeze"
      i. Signs and symptoms
         ➤ Ear pain
         ➤ Tinnitus
         ➤ Dizziness
         ➤ Hearing loss
   2. Nitrogen narcosis, aka "rapture of the deep"
      i. Can occur at bottom of dive.
      ii. Signs and symptoms
         ➤ Altered mentation, impaired judgement
         ➤ Intoxicated sensation, appearance
   3. Decompression sickness, aka "the bends"
      i. Caused by barotrauma during ascent.
      ii. Signs and symptoms
         ➤ Severe pain, especially in the joints and abdomen
         ➤ Altered LOC
         ➤ Dizziness
         ➤ N&V
         ➤ Vertigo
         ➤ Tinnitus

➤ Chest pain

➤ Cough

➤ Pulmonary edema

4. Pulmonary overpressure

   i. Caused by barotrauma during ascent (usually holding breath during ascent).

   ii. Can cause pneumothorax, arterial gas embolism, and pneumomediastinum (abnormal presence of air in the mediastinum).

   iii. Signs and symptoms

   ➤ Chest pain

   ➤ Dyspnea

   ➤ Diminished breath sounds (pneumothorax)

   ➤ Signs and symptoms of stroke (arterial gas embolism)

   ➤ Narrowing pulse pressure (pneumomediastinum)

5. General management of diving emergencies

   i. General management of ALS patients (Patient Assessment chapter) with emphasis on:

   ➤ Administration of high-concentration oxygen.

   ➤ Monitor for signs of pneumothorax.

   ii. Consider continuous positive airway pressure (**not** for pneumothorax).

   iii. Transport to hyperbaric chamber (per local protocol).

   ➤ Use caution with air evacuation due to possible exposure to barometric pressure changes.

VII. HIGH-ALTITUDE SICKNESS

A. Caused by exposure to high-altitude, low-oxygen environments.

B. Acute mountain sickness (AMS)

   1. Typically caused by rapid ascent to about 6,600 feet or above.

Chapter 22

2. Signs and symptoms
   i. Dizziness
   ii. Weakness
   iii. Dyspnea

C. High-altitude cerebral edema (HACE)
   1. Considered severe AMS.
   2. Signs and symptoms
      i. Signs and symptoms of AMS
      ii. Altered mental status
      iii. Ataxia

D. High-altitude pulmonary edema (HAPE)
   1. Signs and symptoms
      i. Dyspnea
      ii. Chest pain
      iii. Cough
      iv. Weakness
      v. Abnormal lung sounds
      vi. Tachypnea
      vii. Tachycardia

E. General management of high-altitude sickness
   1. Halt ascent, descent if possible.
   2. General management of ALS patients (Patient Assessment chapter) with emphasis on high-concentration oxygen administration.
   3. Consider steroids such as dexamethasone per local protocol.

 VIII. LIGHTNING INJURIES

A. High likelihood of respiratory and/or cardiac arrest with VF.

Environmental Emergencies

- **B.** Provide CPR and early defibrillation.

- **C.** Do not triage lightning victims in cardiac arrest as you would other traumatic cardiac arrest patients due to higher survival rates with early CPR and defibrillation.

IX. BITES AND STINGS

- **A.** General management of bites and stings
  1. Ensure scene safety before initiating treatment.
  2. Remove patient from exposure environment.
  3. General management of ALS patients (see Patient Assessment chapter).
  4. Prevent further envenomation when possible, e.g., remove stingers.
  5. Wash area.
  6. Cold compress as indicated for pain.
  7. Assess and manage anaphylaxis as indicated (see Bleeding and Shock chapter).
  8. Contact Poison Control or medical direction for additional guidance as needed.
  9. Transport as indicated.

- **B.** Hymenoptera (wasps, bees, hornets, ants)
  1. Most bites and stings present local problems only, but can induce anaphylactic shock.
  2. Honeybees sting only once, leaving venom sac behind. Other Hymenoptera can sting repeatedly.
  3. Signs and symptoms
     - i. Local pain
     - ii. Redness
     - iii. Swelling
     - iv. Skin welt

C. Spiders
  1. Brown recluse
     i. Bites are not immediately painful and may not be noticed at the time.
     ii. Signs and symptoms
        ➤ Localized pain, redness, and swelling develop over several hours.
        ➤ Local tissue necrosis can develop over days to weeks.
        ➤ In rare cases, fever, chills, N&V, disseminated intravascular coagulation may develop.
     iii. Management
        ➤ General management of ALS patients (see Patient Assessment chapter).
        ➤ No antivenin available.
        ➤ Transport as indicated.
           — *Note:* Antihistamines and surgical repair of necrotic tissue may be necessary.
  2. Black widow
     i. Bites to humans come from female black widow spiders.
     ii. Signs and symptoms
        ➤ Immediate, localized pain, redness, and swelling.
        ➤ Muscle spasms may develop.
        ➤ In rare cases, N&V, seizures, paralysis and decreased LOC.
     iii. Management
        ➤ General management of ALS patients (see Patient Assessment chapter).
           — Monitor carefully for hypertensive crisis.
        ➤ Consider benzodiazepines or calcium gluconate (not calcium chloride) for severe muscle spasms per local protocol.
        ➤ Transport as indicated.
        ➤ *Note:* Antivenin is available.

Environmental Emergencies

- D. Scorpions
    1. Most scorpion stings are unlikely to produce systemic complications.
    2. Signs and symptoms
        - i. Local pain, burning
        - ii. Numbness
        - iii. Slurred speech
        - iv. Hyperactivity (especially in children)
        - v. Nystagmus
        - vi. Muscle twitching
        - vii. Excessive salivation
        - viii. Abdominal cramps, N&V
        - ix. Seizures
    3. Management
        - i. General management of ALS patients (see Patient Assessment chapter).
        - ii. Transport.
        - iii. *Note:* Analgesics may increase toxicity.
        - iv. *Note:* Antivenin (aka antivenom) is available, but there is a high risk of an anaphylactic reaction.
- E. Snakebites
    1. Inappropriate interventions
        - i. Do **not** apply ice, cold packs, etc.
        - ii. Do **not** apply tourniquet.
        - iii. Do **not** incise wound.
        - iv. Do **not** apply electrical stimulation.
        - v. Do **not** use a snake bite kit.
    2. Signs and symptoms of poisonous snake bite
        - i. Local pain, swelling
        - ii. Oozing at the wound site

- iii. Abdominal pain, N&V, diarrhea
- iv. Dizziness, weakness, syncope
- v. Ataxia
- vi. Slurred speech
- vii. Shock
- viii. Circulatory or respiratory failure
- ix. Seizures
- x. *Note:* Onset of symptoms can be rapid, or can be delayed for several hours.

3. General management of snakebites
   - i. General management of ALS patients (see Patient Assessment chapter).
   - ii. Wash wound site.
   - iii. Immobilize bite site (follow local protocol regarding use of constricting bands or compression bandages).
   - iv. Transport to appropriate hospital (consider antivenin availability).

F. Marine animals

1. Includes jellyfish, corals, stingrays, urchins.
2. **All** can cause severe pain and are typically heat sensitive (heat reduces pain).
3. Signs and symptoms
   - i. Intense local pain
   - ii. N&V
   - iii. Dyspnea
   - iv. Weakness
   - v. Tachycardia
   - vi. Hypotension
4. Management
   - i. General management of ALS patients (Patient Assessment chapter).

ii. Follow local protocol regarding use of constricting bands or compression bandages.

iii. Apply heat (110°F–113°F).

REVIEW QUESTIONS
(Answers on pg. 425.)

1. Which of the following is true regarding predisposing risk factors for heat and cold emergencies?
   A. age (pediatric and geriatric patients are at reduced risk)
   B. medications (many medications reduce the risk of heat and cold emergencies
   C. health (chronically ill patients are at an increased risk)
   D. heredity (some people have a familial risk of heat and cold emergencies)

2. Which of the following is a mild to moderate systemic emergency caused by dehydration and electrolyte loss?
   A. heat exhaustion
   B. heat stroke
   C. frostbite
   D. chilblains

3. Which of the following conditions will likely present with decreased LOC, bradycardia, and atrial fibrillation?
   A. mild hypothermia
   B. severe hypothermia
   C. moderate heat exhaustion
   D. heat stroke

Chapter 22

4. Which of the following is recommended for management of patients with a core temperature below 86°F (30°C)?

   A. Discontinue CPR.

   B. Shock VF a maximum of 6 times.

   C. Withhold medications.

   D. Follow standard ACLS guidelines.

5. Your 2-year-old pediatric patient was rescued from the bottom of a swimming pool. The patient is unresponsive with a palpable carotid pulse of 50. You should first:

   A. initiate immediate transport.

   B. obtain IV/IO access.

   C. provide ventilations until the pulse rate is over 100.

   D. begin CPR.

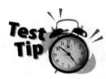

Questions on the certification exam will **not** contain a great deal of irrelevant information. That means two things:

1. What's in the questions is important.

2. Don't "what if" the questions by putting things in that aren't there.

PART VII
SPECIAL PATIENTS

Obstetrical and Gynecological Emergencies

Chapter 23

I. TERMS TO KNOW

A. **Age of fetal viability:** The age at which a human fetus can survive outside the uterus (about 23+ weeks gestation).

B. **Bloody show:** Vaginal discharge of blood and mucus indicating the onset of labor.

C. **Dysmenorrhea:** Normal menstrual cramping.

D. **Fundal height:** Distance in cm from pubic symphysis to top of uterine fundus. Each cm = 1 week of gestation.

E. **Gestational diabetes:** Diabetes diagnosed for the first time during pregnancy.

F. **Gravida:** Total number of pregnancies.

G. **Hyperemesis gravidarum:** Severe nausea and vomiting during pregnancy.

H. **Ketonuria:** Excess ketones (acids) in the urine. Indicates inadequate blood glucose.

I. **Menarche:** First menstrual period during female adolescence.

J. **Menses:** Menstruation.

K. **Mittelschmerz:** Ovulation pain that occurs mid–menstrual cycle.

L. **Multigravida:** A woman who has had at least two pregnancies.

M. **Para:** Total number of pregnancies reaching viable gestational age (live births and stillbirths).

N. **Postpartum:** After delivery.

O. **Premature rupture of membranes (PROM):** Rupture of the amniotic sac prior to the onset of labor.

P. **Primigravida:** A woman who is pregnant for the first time.

Q. **Spontaneous abortion:** Delivery of the fetus prior to 20 weeks gestation; aka miscarriage.

R. **Supine hypotensive syndrome:** Hypotension due to compression of the inferior vena cava and aorta while the mother is supine.

ANATOMY & PHYSIOLOGY REVIEW

> *Note:* See "Respiratory System" in the online Anatomy & Physiology Review at *www.rea.com/paramedic.*

SPECIAL ASSESSMENT CONSIDERATIONS

A. Onset of labor

1. Passage of mucus plug ("bloody show").

2. Rupture of amniotic sac (may not be obvious).

3. Onset of contractions.

B. Determine if delivery is imminent

1. Urge to push.

2. Strong, long, regular contractions about every 2 minutes.

3. *Note:* Check for crowning (during contraction) only if imminent delivery is suspected.

C. Increased risk of injury and death due to motor vehicle collisions, falls, and domestic violence.

D. Determine gestational age of fetus, e.g., how many weeks pregnant, estimated due date, fundal height.

E. Provide emotional support.

F. Carefully monitor for signs of hypoxia, shock, supine hypotensive syndrome.

PATIENT HISTORY

A. Are you pregnant? How many weeks? Due date?

B. Has your water broken? Are you having contractions?

C. Determine GTPAL

 1. **Gravida:** Total number of pregnancies. Twins/triplets count as one. Present pregnancy included.

 2. **Term** births: Number of term deliveries (37+ weeks). Twins/triplets count as one.

 3. **Preterm:** Number of deliveries between 20 and 37 weeks. Twins/triplets count as one. Includes stillbirths.

 4. **Abortions:** Deliveries prior to 20 weeks gestation. Twins/triplets count as one.

 5. **Living** children: Total number of living children.

D. Prenatal care? Any known complications?

E. Are you expecting twins?

F. Vaginal bleeding?

G. Any trauma, including falls, abuse?

> ➤ *Remember:* Homicide is the leading cause of death among pregnant women in the U.S. To learn more, read the Domestic Violence and Pregnancy Fact Sheet published by the National Coalition Against Domestic Violence.

V. OBSTETRICAL COMPLICATIONS

A. Trauma in pregnancy
   1. Pregnant patients at increased risk of injury and death due to motor vehicle accidents, falls, and domestic violence.
   2. Domestic violence during pregnancy
      i. Homicide is the leading cause of death among pregnant women in the U.S.
      ii. Domestic violence during pregnancy is more common than gestational diabetes or preeclampsia; however, most women are not screened for domestic violence or sexual assault.
   3. Any injury to the mother poses risk to the fetus.
      i. Physiological changes during pregnancy can mask the usual signs and symptoms of shock.
      ii. Maintain a high index of suspicion for any pregnant patient that experiences trauma, even in the absence of obvious signs and symptoms of injury, shock, or hypoxia.
      iii. The fetus can be in serious jeopardy even if mother appears uninjured.

B. Hyperemesis
   1. Pathophysiology
      i. Severe vomiting during pregnancy. Occurs in up to 3% of pregnancies.
      ii. Complications include hypovolemia, weight loss, ketonuria.
      iii. Increased risk with multigravida pregnancies.
   2. Management
      i. Protect the patient's airway.
      ii. Intravenous fluids as indicated.
      iii. Antiemetics per local protocol.
      iv. Transport.

Obstetrical and Gynecological Emergencies

> ➤ **Remember:** To avoid supine hypotensive syndrome, do **not** place a pregnant patient supine if she is over 20 weeks gestation. Tilt the mother onto her left side to relieve compression of inferior vena cava and aorta.

- C. Supine hypotensive syndrome
    1. Occurs during third trimester. Weight of gravid uterus and fetus compress inferior vena cava and aorta while mother is supine.
    2. Can cause acute hypotension, nausea, syncope.
    3. Tilt patient on her left side to prevent or correct.
- D. Vaginal bleeding
    1. Common causes
        - i. Spontaneous abortion (miscarriage)
        - ii. Ectopic pregnancy
        - iii. Abruptio placenta
        - iv. Placenta previa
        - v. Postpartum hemorrhage (under 500 mL is normal)
    2. General management of obstetrics (OB)-related vaginal bleeding
        - i. General management of advanced life support (ALS) patients (Patient Assessment chapter).
        - ii. Treat for shock as indicated.
        - iii. Consider postpartum interventions, per local protocol:
            - ➤ Fundal massage.
            - ➤ Breastfeeding.
            - ➤ Oxytocin administration.
        - iv. Rapid transport to appropriate facility.
- E. Premature rupture of membranes (PROM)
    1. Pathophysiology
        - i. Rupture of membranes prior to 37 weeks gestation (about 8% of pregnancies).

Chapter 23

        ii. Risk factors include trauma, a previous history of PROM, short cervical length, vaginal bleeding, smoking, drug use, malnutrition.

    2. Assessment and management

        i. History of present illness? Leakage of amniotic fluid? Trauma? Fetal movement? Vaginal bleeding?

        ii. Transport to appropriate facility.

F. Uterine rupture

    1. Can result from labor or trauma.

    2. Signs and symptoms

        i. Severe abdominal pain

        ii. Signs and symptoms of shock

        iii. Possible absence of fetal heart tones

    3. Management

        i. General management of ALS patients (Patient Assessment chapter).

        ii. Treat for shock.

        iii. Rapid transport (for mother and to determine fetus viability).

G. Spontaneous abortion (miscarriage)

    1. Delivery of fetus before 20 weeks of gestation.

    2. More appropriately referred to as "early loss of pregnancy."

    3. Signs and symptoms

        i. Severe, intermittent cramping, lower abdominal pain

        ii. Vaginal bleeding

        iii. Passage of tissue, clots

    4. Management

        i. General management of ALS patients (see Patient Assessment chapter).

        ii. Treat for shock.

        iii. Emotional support.

        iv. Rapid transport.

Obstetrical and Gynecological Emergencies

- H. Placenta previa
    1. Abnormal placement of placenta over cervical opening.
    2. Typically occurs late in second or third trimester.
    3. Signs and symptoms
        i. Bright red, painless vaginal bleeding late in pregnancy
        ii. *Note:* Treat painless vaginal bleeding during later stages of pregnancy as placenta previa until proven otherwise.
    4. Management
        i. General management of ALS patients (see Patient Assessment chapter).
        ii. Treat for shock as indicated.
        iii. Transport for possible cesarean section.
- I. Abruptio placenta
    1. Premature separation of the placenta from the uterine wall, causing intrauterine hemorrhage.
    2. Typically occurs during third trimester.
    3. High risk of fetal mortality.
    4. Signs and symptoms
        i. Lower abdominal pain and vaginal bleeding (blood loss can be trapped, with no evident vaginal bleeding).
        ii. Signs and symptoms of shock with or without vaginal bleeding.
        iii. Risk factors include trauma, maternal hypertension, maternal drug use.
    5. Management
        i. Aggressive management of shock.
        ii. Place patient left lateral recumbent.
        iii. Rapid transport to appropriate facility.
- J. Hypertensive complications of pregnancy
    1. Preeclampsia
        i. Pathophysiology
            ➤ Most common hypertensive disorder of pregnancy.

- Can progress from mild to severe.
- Increase in systolic pressure of 30 mmHg and/or 5 mmHg increase in diastolic pressure on at least two occasions (at least 6 hrs apart).
- Usually occurs from last 10 weeks of gestation through 48 hrs postpartum.

  ii. Signs and symptoms
- Hypertension
- Edema
- Headache
- Visual disturbances
- Hyperactive reflexes
- Pulmonary edema
- Increased urinary output

  iii. Management
- General management of ALS patients (see Patient Assessment chapter).
- Keep patient calm, dim lights, avoid lights and siren.
- Place left lateral recumbent.
- Consider magnesium sulfate per local protocol.

2. Eclampsia
  i. Seizures due to hypertensive disorder of pregnancy.
  ii. High risk of maternal and fetal death.
  iii. Signs and symptoms
- Generalized tonic-clonic seizures
- History of preeclampsia
- Preceded by signs and symptoms of preeclampsia

  iv. Management
- Same as above.
- Magnesium sulfate preferred to control seizures, then diazepam or other benzodiazepines.

Obstetrical and Gynecological Emergencies

- **K.** Supine hypotensive syndrome
    1. Occurs in later stages of pregnancy when uterus compresses inferior vena cava while supine.
    2. Signs and symptoms
        - i. Patient supine for extended period
        - ii. Dizziness
        - iii. Syncope
        - iv. Hypotension
    3. Management
        - i. Place patient left lateral recumbent (usually sufficient).
        - ii. Treat for shock if not resolved with repositioning.

- **L.** Pulmonary embolism
    1. Can occur anytime during or shortly after pregnancy.
    2. Signs and symptoms
        - i. Acute-onset dyspnea
        - ii. Chest pain
    3. Management
        - i. General management of ALS patients (Patient Assessment chapter).
        - ii. Rapid transport.

- **M.** Maternal cardiac arrest
    1. Attempt to determine gestational age.
    2. Begin CPR per current American Heart Association (AHA) Basic Life Support guidelines.
        - i. Do **not** use mechanical CPR devices for maternal cardiac arrest patients.
    3. Manually displace uterus off aorta and vena cava (push uterus to the left).
        - i. Effective chest compressions can be performed with patients tilted on their left side up to 30 degrees.
        - ii. Use a pillow, blanket, etc., to wedge patient onto her left side.

4. Defibrillate VF and PVT per current AHA Advanced Cardiovascular Life Support (ACLS) guidelines.

5. Provide rapid airway management and ventilation with 100% oxygen (**no** hyperventilation).

6. Administer emergency drugs per current AHA ACLS guidelines.

7. Transport to appropriate hospital with perimortem cesarean capability.

STAGES OF LABOR

A. First stage

1. Begins with the onset of contractions and ends with full cervical dilation.

2. The cervix is fully dilated at 10 cm, allowing infant's head to enter the birth canal.

3. Contractions initially occur at widespread intervals and become more severe and closer together over time.

4. The mucus plug (and some blood) that seals the uterine opening passes; aka "bloody show."

5. The amniotic sac may rupture spontaneously.

6. Stage one typically lasts longer for first-time pregnancies.

B. Second stage

1. Begins with full cervical dilation and ends with delivery of the baby.

2. Contractions are close together.

3. Mother feels intense pressure and urge to push.

C. Third stage

1. Begins once baby is delivered and ends with delivery of the placenta.

2. Placenta typically delivers within 30 minutes after delivery of the baby.

3. There will be an increase in vaginal bleeding shortly before the placenta delivers and the mother will feel the urge to push again.

Obstetrical and Gynecological Emergencies

D. Stage one: From the onset of labor through full cervical dilation

E. Stage two: From full cervical dilation through delivery of the newborn

F. Stage three: From delivery of newborn through delivery of the placenta

G. Stage four: Recovery of the mother

VII. TRANSPORT OR DELIVER

A. Transport the mother to the hospital for delivery whenever possible.

B. If delivery is imminent (crowning, urge to push), then prepare to deliver on scene.

C. When in doubt, consult medical control.

D. Imminent delivery indications

1. The mother has strong, frequent contractions under 2 minutes apart with little break between contractions. *Note:* Contractions are timed from the beginning of one contraction to the beginning of the next contraction.
2. The abdomen is rigid during contractions.
3. The mother feels the urge to push.
4. Mother may report passage of mucus plug and/or rupture of the amniotic sac.
5. Crowning
   i. Crowning is the appearance of the baby's head in the birth canal.
   ii. Assess for crowning if you suspect imminent delivery.

VIII. NORMAL FIELD DELIVERY

A. Prepare OB kit.

B. Position mother (not supine).

Chapter 23

C. Assess for crowning.

D. If necessary, manually rupture amniotic sac to facilitate delivery.

E. Assess for presence of thick meconium in amniotic fluid.

F. Support head, guide external rotation (avoid fontanelles).

G. Ensure cord is not around baby's neck.

H. Guide presenting shoulder up, then guide down to facilitate delivery.

I. Begin newborn assessment and interventions as indicated.

J. Clamp and cut cord once done pulsating.

K. Make transport decision while awaiting placental delivery.

L. Prepare for delivery of placenta. Gently guide, do not pull.

M. Monitor postpartum hemorrhage, signs of shock.

N. Uterine massage and/or breastfeeding can reduce postpartum hemorrhage.

O. Transport mother, baby, and placenta.

IX. NEWBORN CARE/NEONATAL RESUSCITATION

A. Routine suctioning of the neonate is **not** recommended.

B. See Neonatology chapter for additional information about newborn assessment and resuscitation.

X. ABNORMAL DELIVERY COMPLICATIONS

A. Breech presentation
1. Either both feet or buttocks present first in birth canal.

Obstetrical and Gynecological Emergencies

2. Management
    i. Transport rapidly if possible for possible cesarean.
    ii. Support baby during delivery.
    iii. If head becomes trapped, form a "V" with fingers in birth canal over baby's face to facilitate breathing.

B. Prolapsed cord
   1. Umbilical cord is presenting part.
   2. Cord can become compressed during delivery, shutting down fetal circulation.
   3. Management
       i. Do **not** attempt delivery.
       ii. Use gloved hand to gently ease fetus off the cord.
       iii. Place mother in knee-chest position.
       iv. Transport immediately to appropriate facility.

C. Limb presentation
   1. Arm or leg is presenting part.
   2. Do **not** attempt delivery.
   3. Place mother in knee-chest position.
   4. Cover limb to prevent heat loss.
   5. Transport immediately for cesarean.

D. Nuchal cord
   1. Cord is wrapped around baby's neck.
   2. Management
       i. Gently slip cord over baby's head (this usually works).
       ii. **Only** if cord compression occurs and unable to slip cord over baby's head: Clamp the cord in two places (2" apart) and cut.
       iii. *Note:* Determine possibility of multiple births before making decision to cut umbilical cord.

E. Multiple births
   1. Increased risk of preterm labor and low-birth-weight hypothermia.
   2. Request additional resources and prepare additional equipment.
   3. May be one shared or two separate placentas.

F. Meconium
   1. Presence of fetal stool in amniotic fluid.
   2. Appears as thick light yellow to green "pea soup"–colored amniotic fluid.
   3. Indicates likelihood of fetal hypoxia.
   4. Increased risk of aspiration and infection.
   5. Management
      i. No intervention needed for light meconium staining.
      ii. For thick meconium, suction the neonate's airway as able to reduce aspiration risk.
      iii. Consider use of endotracheal tube and meconium aspirator attached to suction, per local protocol.

> *Remember:* The pregnant patient is at risk of developing hypoxia rapidly. Monitor breathing status and SpO_2 carefully. When in doubt, administer oxygen.

XI. GYNECOLOGICAL EMERGENCIES

A. Ectopic pregnancy
   1. Pregnancy where the fertilized egg implants outside of the uterus, usually the fallopian tubes.
   2. Occurs during the first trimester. Patient may not know she is pregnant.
   3. A ruptured fallopian tube will cause massive hemorrhage.
   4. Requires rapid surgical intervention.

5. Signs and symptoms
   i. Diffuse abdominal tenderness progressing to sharp, localized, unilateral lower quadrant abdominal pain (may radiate to shoulder)
   ii. Late or missed menstrual cycle
   iii. Syncope
   iv. Vaginal bleeding
   v. Signs and symptoms of shock
   vi. *Note:* Encourage transport for any female patient of childbearing years with abdominal pain for suspected ectopic pregnancy.

B. Pelvic inflammatory disease (PID)
   1. Infection of female reproductive tract, including gonorrhea and chlamydia.
   2. Can be acute or chronic and lead to infertility, ectopic pregnancy, and sepsis.
   3. Signs and symptoms
      i. Diffuse lower abdominal pain
      ii. Increased pain with intercourse or walking
      iii. Fever, chills
      iv. N&V
      v. Foul-smelling vaginal discharge
      vi. Mid-cycle vaginal bleeding

C. Ovarian cyst
   1. Fluid-filled pockets in the ovary that can rupture.
   2. Signs and symptoms
      i. Severe unilateral abdominal pain
      ii. Vaginal bleeding

D. Endometriosis
1. Disorder causing uterine tissue to develop outside of the uterus.
2. Signs and symptoms
   i. Dull, cramping pelvic or lower abdominal pain
   ii. Abnormal menstrual bleeding

E. Sexual assault
1. Victims of sexual assault can be male or female, young or old. Patients are often females with possible gynecologic trauma.
2. First priority is patient care, then reporting to appropriate authorities, e.g., law enforcement, child or adult protective services.
3. Guidelines for management of sexual assault victims
   i. Treat patient first, preserve evidence second.
   ii. Provide psychological support.
   iii. Provide same-sex EMS provider when possible.
   iv. Do not disrupt possible crime scene any more than necessary.
   v. Handle clothing as little as possible.
   vi. Place any clothing or bloody items that have been removed in *brown paper bags*.
   vii. Do not cut through tears or holes in clothing.
   viii. Only examine perineal area if necessary to manage significant injury.
   ix. Encourage patient not to change clothes, shower, urinate, or douche prior to medical examination at hospital.

F. General management of gynecological patients
1. General management of ALS patients (Patient Assessment chapter).
2. Treat for shock as indicated.
3. Remember, you should consider ectopic pregnancy for any female patient of childbearing years with abdominal pain.

REVIEW QUESTIONS
(Answers on pg. 425.)

1. Which of the following is included as part of the "GTPAL" assessment?
   A. abortions
   B. GCS score
   C. prenatal care
   D. last oral intake

2. Which of the following is the leading cause of death among pregnant women in the U.S.?
   A. homicide
   B. suicide
   C. pulmonary embolism
   D. eclamptic seizures

3. Which of the following is recommended to prevent supine hypotensive syndrome in the pregnant patient?
   A. IV fluid bolus.
   B. Place the mother in the Trendelenburg position.
   C. Tilt the mother to her left side.
   D. Apply gentle posterior pressure to the uterus.

4. Which of the following indicates that delivery is imminent?
   A. crowning
   B. rupture of membranes
   C. contractions every 2 minutes
   D. at least 39 weeks gestation

Chapter 23

5. Your patient is 36 weeks pregnant. She complains of painless vaginal bleeding. You should suspect:

   A. ectopic pregnancy.

   B. abruptio placenta.

   C. placenta previa.

   D. spontaneous abortion.

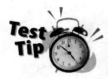

You will not likely see many questions with "all of the above" or "none of the above" answer choices (that's good!). Use caution with any questions that include "except." Unlike most questions, "except" questions usually have *three correct* answer choices and *one incorrect* choice. You are looking for the **incorrect** choice. Slow down and read these questions carefully.

Chapter 24

Neonatology

I. TERMS TO KNOW

A. **Acrocyanosis:** Cyanosis of the hands and feet due to poor perfusion.

B. **Gestation:** Time from conception to birth.

C. **Meconium:** Fetal material in amniotic fluid from baby's first bowel movement.

D. **Neonate:** Newborns from birth to 1 month old.

E. **Patent ductus arteriosus:** Ductus arteriosus fails to close during embryonic development, causing aortic blood flow into pulmonary artery.

F. **Preterm:** Infant delivered prior to 37 weeks gestation.

G. **Spina bifida:** Birth defect that occurs when the spine and spinal cord don't form properly.

II. PATHOPHYSIOLOGY

A. Risk factors for newborn complications

1. Multiple gestation pregnancies
2. No prenatal care
3. Mother under 16 or over 35 years of age
4. Drug or alcohol abuse during pregnancy
5. Preterm labor
6. Meconium

Chapter 24

7. Amniotic sac rupture more than 24 hours prior to delivery
8. Abnormal presentation during delivery
9. Prolonged labor or explosive delivery

B. Resuscitation
1. About 10% of newborns require assistance to begin breathing.
2. About 1% require full resuscitative measures.
3. Need for resuscitation inversely related to birth weight (about 80% of newborns under 3.5 lb require resuscitation).
4. Cardiac arrest in neonates usually due to hypoxia.

III. CONGENITAL ANOMALIES

A. A leading cause of death among infants.

B. Congenital heart defects
1. May increase pulmonary flow, causing congestive heart failure.
2. May decrease pulmonary flow, compromising oxygenation.
3. May obstruct blood flow.

C. Diaphragmatic hernia
1. Abdominal contents enter thorax through opening in diaphragm (rare).
2. Signs and symptoms
    i. Dyspnea and cyanosis unresponsive to oxygenation and ventilation
    ii. Bowel sounds auscultated in the chest
    iii. Flat abdomen
3. Management
    i. Position head and thorax above abdomen.
    ii. Insert orogastric (OG) or nasogastric (NG) tube with low, intermittent suction (facilitates improved ventilation).

iii. Do **not** initiate bag-valve-mask (BVM) ventilation without intubation (increases gastric distention). Intubate if BVM ventilations are necessary.

iv. Rapid transport for surgical repair.

D. Spina bifida

1. Spinal cord is exposed.

i. Cover with moist, sterile, occlusive dressing and place newborn in prone or lateral position.

> *Remember:* Visit *https://cpr.heart.org/en/resuscitation-science/cpr-and-ecc-guidelines/algorithms* to view the American Heart Association's Neonatal Resuscitation Algorithm.

> *Remember:*
> 1. Delayed cord clamping can improve the newborn's condition, especially in preterm infants.
> 2. Tachycardia in newborns = adequate oxygenation.
> 3. Avoid 100% oxygen during resuscitation of newborns due to increased risk of mortality. 21% oxygen is appropriate for a term newborn.
> 4. Perform chest compressions on newborns only after providing adequate ventilations first.
>
> — *Circulation* 2019;140(24):e922–e930
> — *Resuscitation* 2021;161:291–326

IV. NEWBORN ASSESSMENT AND RESUSCITATION

A. Routine delivery (term newborn, good muscle tone, breathing adequately)

1. Routine care: Keep warm and dry, clear secretions as indicated.
2. See Table 24-1: Normal Assessment Findings in Newborns

Chapter 24

Normal Vitals	Normal Blood Glucose
➤ Respirations: 40–60/min ➤ Pulse: 100–180/min **Normal SpO$_2$** ➤ At least 93% **Normal Temp** ➤ 98–100 degrees F (36.7–37.8° C)	➤ At least 45 mg/dL **Normal Weight** ➤ About 5½–8½ lbs **Normal APGAR** ➤ 7–10

Figure 24-1. Normal Assessment Findings in Newborns

B. **Not** routine delivery (not term, underweight, poor muscle tone, not breathing adequately). **Hint:** Refer to current American Heart Association (AHA) Neonatal Resuscitation Algorithm, available online.

1. Dry, warm, position, suction, tactile stimulation.
2. Check respirations and heart rate.
    i. If breathing adequately and heart rate over 100:
        ➤ Check skin color.
        ➤ Monitor SpO$_2$, administer blow-by oxygen as indicated. *Note:* see Table 24-1: Anticipated Pulse Oximetry in Newborns Over Time.

Anticipated Pulse Oximetry in Newborns over Time

Time Since Birth	Anticipated Pulse Oximetry
1 minute	60%–65%
3 minutes	70%–75%
5 minutes	80%–85%
10 minutes	85%–90%

Table 24-1. NASEMCO National Model EMS Clinical Guidelines

3. If apneic/gasping breaths or heart rate below 100:
    i. Begin BVM ventilations.
        ➤ *Note:* Newborns frequently need higher pressures for initial ventilations. Disable pop-off valve on BVM for initial ventilations, then enable if continued positive pressure ventilation (PPV) is needed.
    ii. Monitor SpO_2/ECG monitoring.
    iii. *Note:* All above interventions should not take longer than 1 minute!
4. Check heart rate
    i. If heart rate is 100 or more, provide supportive care.
    ii. Heart rate below 100:
        ➤ Ensure adequate PPV and recheck heart rate.
        ➤ Heart rate below 60:
            — Intubate.
            — Begin CPR (3:1 compressions: ventilations).
            — Ensure adequate BVM ventilation.
            — Reassess heart rate.
            — If below 60, intravenous (IV) epinephrine, assess for hypovolemia, pneumothorax.
        ➤ Heart rate 60–99:
            — Continue BVM ventilation with high-concentration oxygen.
        ➤ Heart rate 100 or more:
            — Supportive care.

C. Apgar scoring (see Table 24-2)
   1. Assess Apgar at 1 minute and 5 minutes post delivery.
   2. *Note:* Do **not** delay critical interventions for newborns to obtain an Apgar score. Apgar scores are **not** necessary to guide resuscitation efforts.

Chapter 24

APGAR Scoring (0–10)		
Appearance (skin)	Pink (everywhere)	2
	Pink (core only)	1
	Cyanosis (central)	0
Pulse (rate)	Over 100+/min	2
	60–99	1
	Less than 60	0
Grimace (irritability)	Crying	2
	Grimacing	1
	No response	0
Activity (muscle tone)	Active	2
	Some motion	1
	Limp	0
Respirations (effort)	Strong cry	2
	Slow or irregular	1
	Absent	0
7–10: likely only routine care needed 4–6: likely stimulation/oxygenation needed 0–3: Begin resuscitation immediately.		

Table 24-2. APGAR Scoring (0–10)

- **D.** Special considerations
    1. Bulb syringe
        - i. Routine suctioning with bulb syringe **no longer recommended** (can stimulate the vagus nerve, causing bradycardia and hypoxia).
    2. Suction
        - i. If amniotic fluid is clear, do not suction unless airway is obstructed or BVM is required.
    3. Meconium
        - i. For thick meconium in nonvigorous newborns, quickly clear airway and initiate ventilations within 1 minute of delivery (before stimulating to breathe).
        - ii. Use endotracheal tube (ETT) connected to meconium aspirator to suction trachea (100 cmH$_2$O of suction or less) per local protocol.

iii. Do not intubate with contaminated ETT; use a new one.

iv. Quickly oxygenate and ventilate as indicated. *Note:* Suctioning can increase hypoxia and should be completed quickly.

4. Gastric decompression (OG/NG tube) indicated for newborns with gastric distention (often due to prolonged BVM ventilation).

5. Medication administration

   i. Consider umbilical vein or intraosseous (IO) for vascular access for medications. *Note:* You must ensure that no air is administered via an umbilical catheter.

   ii. Epinephrine administration per current advanced American Heart Association guidelines.

   iii. Naloxone **not indicated** in newborn resuscitation (can cause withdrawal symptoms).

   iv. If IV fluids indicated, administer 10 mL/kg of normal saline or lactated Ringer's.

   v. If dextrose indicated for hypoglycemia (below 45 mg/dL), use 10% dextrose solution (D10, **not** D50).

E. Cutting the cord

1. There is no urgency to clamp and cut the cord **unless** resuscitation measures are needed.

2. Delayed cord clamping acceptable for vigorous newborns who are adequately breathing and crying.

3. Place one clamp about 4" from newborn and another clamp 2" further and cut between clamps.

V. NEONATAL EMERGENCIES

A. Bradycardia

1. The primary cause of bradycardia in pediatric patients (including newborns) is hypoxia.

2. **Always** manage a bradycardic newborn/infant/pediatric patient for hypoxia first, then consider other causes, e.g., increased intracranial pressure, cardiac anomalies, metabolic problem, medications, etc.

3. **Remember:** Begin CPR for any unresponsive pediatric patient with a pulse below 60 beats per minute.

B. Premature newborn
   1. Newborn delivered prior to 37 weeks gestation.
   2. Increased risk of:
      i. Underweight newborn (under about 5.5 lb).
      ii. Respiratory compromise.
      iii. Hypothermia.
      iv. Head bleeds.
   3. Management
      i. Treat as regular newborn.
      ii. Resuscitate as indicated per AHA guidelines.
      iii. Manage hypoxia and hypothermia as indicated.
      iv. Rapid transport to appropriate facility.

C. Hypovolemia
   1. Leading cause of shock in newborns.
      i. Dehydration (diarrhea, vomiting, fever) most common cause.
      ii. Hemorrhage.
      iii. Third spacing of fluids.
   2. Signs and symptoms
      i. Pale, cool skin
      ii. Weak or absent peripheral pulses
      iii. Delayed capillary refill (not associated with hypothermia)
      iv. Decreased level of consciousness
      v. Decreased urinary output (dark urine or dry diaper)
   3. Management
      i. IV/IO fluids (normal saline or lactated Ringer's) at 10 mL/kg over 5–10 minutes and reassess.
      ii. Repeat as indicated (40–60 mL/kg may be needed).

D. Seizures
   1. Generalized tonic-clonic seizures rare in neonates; instead they are usually:
      i. Subtle seizures with apnea and swim or pedal-like movements.
      ii. Tonic (rigid) seizures.
      iii. Focal clonic seizures.
      iv. Myoclonic seizures (brief focal or generalized jerking of extremities).
   2. Common causes of neonatal seizures
      i. Seizures in newborns suggestive of neurological disorder
      ii. Hypoglycemia (blood glucose below 45 mg/dL)
      iii. Sepsis
      iv. Fever
      v. Meningitis
      vi. Medication withdrawal
   3. Management
      i. General management of advanced life support (ALS) patients (Patient Assessment chapter).
      ii. Anticonvulsant meds per local protocol.
      iii. Dextrose (D10) for hypoglycemia.
      iv. Rapid transport.

E. Fever
   1. Normal newborn temp: 99.5°F (37.5°C).
   2. Rectal temp of 100.4°F (38°C) is considered febrile.
      i. Oral temp about 1°F below rectal.
      ii. Axillary temp about 2°F below rectal.
   3. Any neonate with a fever should be treated for possible sepsis or meningitis.
   4. Do **not** apply cold packs.
   5. Transport.

F. Neonatal jaundice
   1. Usually due to excess bilirubin caused by liver immaturity.
   2. Can last 1–2 weeks after delivery.
   3. Usually treated successfully by phototherapy (blue spectrum light).

REVIEW QUESTIONS
(Answers on pg. 426.)

1. What percentage of newborns require assistance to start breathing?
   A. about 10%
   B. about 1%
   C. about 50%
   D. about 90%

2. Your newborn patient has dyspnea and cyanosis that is unresponsive to oxygenation and ventilation. You auscultate bowel sounds in the chest. You should suspect:
   A. hiatal hernia.
   B. diaphragmatic hernia.
   C. bowel obstruction.
   D. congenital heart defect.

3. You have just dried, warmed, and positioned a newborn. The newborn has a pulse rate of 50. You should immediately:
   A. provide ventilations and reassess heart rate.
   B. begin chest compressions.
   C. administer blow-by oxygen.
   D. obtain an Apgar score.

Neonatology

4. What is the correct compression to ventilation ratio for a newborn in cardiac arrest?

    A. 15:2
    B. 30:2
    C. 5:1
    D. 3:1

5. Which of the following regarding newborn resuscitation is correct?

    A. Immediately clamp and cut the cord following delivery.
    B. Begin chest compressions if the heart rate is below 100.
    C. Routine suctioning with a bulb syringe is not recommended.
    D. Dextrose 10% is recommended for a blood glucose below 70 mg/dL.

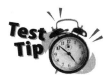

The test will end for one of three reasons:

1. Because you passed (you!) or failed (not you!)
2. Because time is up (over 99% of candidates finish the exam in the time allowed).
3. Because you reached the maximum number of questions. Paramedic candidates will see between 80 and 150 questions.

Pediatrics

Chapter 25

I. TERMS TO KNOW

A. **ALTE:** Apparent life-threatening event.

B. **BRUE:** Brief, resolved, unexplained event.

C. **Mottling/mottled:** Abnormal skin coloring due to vasoconstriction and poor circulation.

D. **Neglect:** Failure of caregiver to provide basic necessities.

E. **Petechiae:** Small, purple, nonblanching spots on skin.

F. **Respiratory arrest:** Apnea.

G. **Respiratory distress:** Increased rate and effort of breathing.

H. **Respiratory failure:** Inadequate oxygenation and ventilation.

I. **SIDS:** Sudden infant death syndrome.

J. **SUID:** Sudden unexplained infant death.

K. **Tenting:** Poor skin turgor (slow retraction of skin after being pinched), indicating possible dehydration.

II. DEVELOPMENTAL STAGES AND NORMAL VITALS

A. See Normal Vital Signs and Developmental Characteristics tables (Tables 25-1 and 25-2).

Table 25-1: Normal Vital Signs

Age	Pulse-Awake (beats/minute)	Pulse-Sleeping (beats/minute)	Respiratory Rate (breaths/minute)	Systolic BP (mmHg)
Preterm less than 1 kg	120–150		30–60	39–59
Preterm 1–3 kg	120–160		30–60	60–75
Newborn	100–205	85–160	30–60	67–84
Up to 1 year	100–190	90–160	30–60	72–104
1–2 years	100–190	90–160	24–40	86–106
2–3 years	98–140	60–120	24–40	86–106
3–4 years	80–140	60–100	24–40	89–112
4–5 years	80–140	60–100	22–34	89–112
5–6 years	75–140	58–90	22–34	89–112
6–10 years	75–140	58–90	18–30	97–115
10–12 years	75–118	58–90	18–30	102–120
12–13 years	60–100	58–90	15–20	110–131
13–15 years	60–100	50–90	15–20	110–131
15 years or older	60–100	50–90	15–20	110–131

Source: Extrapolated from the 2020 American Heart Association Pediatric Advanced Life Support tables from the Nursing Care of the Critically Ill Child, and from web Box 1: Existing reference ranges for respiratory rate and heart rate in the appendix of the article by Fleming, et al., published in Lancet.

Note: While many factors affect blood pressure (e.g., pain, activity, hydration), it is imperative to rapidly recognize hypotension, especially in children. For children of the ages 1–10, hypotension is present if the systolic blood pressure is less than 70 mmHg + (child's age in years x 2) mmHg.

Table 25-2: Developmental Characteristics

	Physical Development	Cognitive Development
Birth to 6 months	• Turns head/controls gaze • Recognizes caregivers (2–6 months) • Makes eye contact (2–6 months) • Rolls over (2–6 months)	• Communicates by crying • Trust develops • Increased awareness of surroundings (2–6 months) • Seeks attention (2–6 months)
6–12 months	• Can sit/crawl • Puts anything in mouth • Teething	• Babbles • Object curiosity • Separation anxiety/tantrums
12–18 months	• Crawls/walks • Sensory development	• Imitates • Understands "make-believe" • Begins developing vocabulary • Separation anxiety
18–24 months	• Runs/climbs • Good balance	• Understands cause/effect • Vocabulary improves • Object attachment
Preschool	• Physically active	• Highly verbal and literal • Can set goals • Monster fear • Can feel guilt
School Age	• Approaching adult anatomy • Breast development/onset of menstrual cycle in females	• Analytical • Peer/popularity concerns

III. ANATOMY & PHYSIOLOGY REVIEW

Note: See "Respiratory System" in the online Anatomy & Physiology Review at *www.rea.com/paramedic*.

IV. PATHOPHYSIOLOGY

A. About one in five pediatric deaths is due to trauma.

B. Motor vehicle accidents are the leading cause of traumatic injury deaths in pediatrics.

C. Respiratory problems, such as bronchiolitis, are the leading cause of pediatric hospitalizations.

D. Bradycardia = hypoxia until proven otherwise.

E. Hypotension is a **late** sign of shock. Do **not** wait for hypotension to treat for suspected hypovolemia/shock.

> *Remember:* Bradycardia in pediatric patients should **always** be regarded as a sign of hypoxia until proven otherwise.

V. PEDIATRIC ASSESSMENT TRIANGLE (PAT)

A. Used to quickly inform general impression: sick or not sick/hurt or not hurt.

B. Intended to be a visual and auditory assessment that can be completed before stressing a child with a hands-on assessment.

C. An abnormal finding in any of the three components of PAT can indicate need for rapid stabilization and rapid transport.

D. The ABCs of the PAT
   1. **Appearance** (mental status and muscle tone) "TICLS"
      i. **Tone:** Assess for movement, muscle tone, listlessness.

ii. **Interactivity:** Assess for alertness, reactivity to stimulus, interaction with the environment.

iii. **Consolability:** Can the child be consoled by the parents or caregivers?

iv. **Look/gaze:** Is the child able to fix their gaze, or do they appear "out of it"?

v. **Speech/cry:** Assess speech in older children or strength of cry in younger children/infants.

vi. *Note:* Abnormalities in appearance may indicate central nervous system (CNS) problem, e.g., altered level of consciousness (LOC), seizures, toxicology, diabetic problem, etc.

2. Work of **Breathing** (respiratory rate and effort)

   i. Accessory muscle use/retractions/flaring.

   ii. Abnormal airway sounds.

   iii. Posturing/tripod breathing.

   iv. After PAT: Auscultate lung sounds.

   v. *Note:* Abnormalities in work of breathing may indicate respiratory problem (trauma or medical).

3. **Circulation** to skin (skin color)

   i. Skin color (normal, pale, mottled, cyanotic)

   ii. After PAT

   ➤ Capillary refill

   ➤ Central vs. peripheral pulses

   ➤ Temperature

   iii. *Note:* Abnormalities here may indicate shock (trauma or medical).

E. Use PAT to help determine transport priority.

1. Urgent: Manage immediate life threats (primary and rapid secondary) and transport immediately.

2. Nonurgent: Can complete secondary assessment on scene prior to transport.

Chapter 25

VI. PEDIATRIC ASSESSMENT TIPS

A. Tachypnea is an early sign of respiratory distress.

B. A slowing respiratory rate may indicate impending respiratory failure.

C. Nasal flaring is a sign of respiratory distress.

D. Cyanosis in mucous membranes and nail beds is a late sign of respiratory failure.

E. Cyanosis of the extremities only indicates shock.

F. Capillary refill is a reliable sign of perfusion only in patients under 6 years of age.
   1. *Note:* Capillary refill over 2 seconds indicates poor perfusion.

G. Maintain high index of suspicion for dehydration (vomiting, diarrhea, dry diapers, skin tenting, poor circulation, etc.).

H. Altered LOC (e.g., inconsolable or unable to recognize parents) may indicate poor CNS perfusion.

I. Bradycardia, especially in a distressed infant or pediatric patient, likely indicates impending cardiac arrest.

J. Strong peripheral pulses indicate adequate perfusion.

K. Decreased peripheral perfusion is an early indication of shock.

VII. RISK FACTORS FOR IMPENDING CARDIAC ARREST

A. Respirations over 60 per minute.

B. Pulse rate under 80 or over 180 (patients under 5 years of age).

C. Respiratory distress.

D. Trauma or burn injuries.

E. Cyanosis.

F. Altered LOC.

G. Seizures.

H. Fever with petechiae.

I. *Note:* Cardiac arrest in pediatric patients is usually caused by respiratory failure or shock.

VIII. PEDIATRIC MANAGEMENT TIPS

A. Basic airway management

1. Use oropharyngeal airway device (OPA) only for unresponsive patients without gag reflex.

2. Insert with use of a tongue blade.

3. Do **not** insert OPA with 180-degree rotation as with adults

4. Do **not** use nasopharyngeal airway device (NPA) on patients with suspected face or head trauma.

5. Size OPAs and NPAs as with adults.

6. Decrease suction pressure (max 100 mmHg in infants).

7. Decrease suction time to reduce hypoxia.

B. Advanced airway management

1. *Tip:* Use resuscitation tape, length-based tape app, or card for appropriate tube size, depth, etc.

2. Calculating pediatric endotracheal tube (ETT) size: (16 + age in years) ÷ 4.

3. Verify proper ETT placement: See Airway/Oxygenation/Ventilation chapter.

C. Ventilation

1. Avoid hyperventilation during BVM ventilation.

2. Utilize waveform capnography when available.

Chapter 25

3. Do **not** use flow-restricted, oxygen-powered ventilatory device on pediatric patients.
4. Avoid BVM devices with pop-off valves.
5. Insert orogastric or nasogastric tube as indicated for gastric decompression.

IX. SPECIFIC PEDIATRIC EMERGENCIES

A. See previous chapters for the following:
   1. Asthma: See Pulmonology chapter.
   2. Croup: See Airway/Oxygenation/Ventilation chapter.
   3. Drowning: See Environmental Emergencies chapter
   4. Diabetes: See Endocrinology chapter.
   5. Meningitis: See Hematology chapter.
   6. Pneumonia: See Pulmonology chapter.
   7. Poisoning/overdose: See Toxicology chapter.
   8. Seizures: See Neurology chapter.

B. Bronchopulmonary dysplasia
   1. Chronic lung disease that typically affects premature newborns and infants.
   2. Bronchi and alveoli damaged in the neonatal period, often due to positive pressure ventilation (PPV) and high-concentration oxygen.
   3. Causes recurrent respiratory infections and exercise-induced bronchospasm.
   4. Management may include inhaled bronchodilators, continuous positive airway pressure, and PPV as indicated.

C. Epiglottitis
   1. Acute infection/inflammation of the epiglottis.
   2. Rare, but potentially life-threatening due to airway obstruction.
   3. Signs and symptoms
      i. Acute-onset fever and cough
      ii. Sore throat

iii. Dyspnea

iv. Stridor

v. Drooling

vi. Tripod breathing

vii. Accessory muscle use

4. Management

   i. Do **not** aggravate child (may worsen airway compromise).

   ➤ Do **not** visualize airway, force suction, start prophylactic IV, etc.

   ii. Supplemental oxygen as tolerated by patient.

   iii. Consider nebulized epinephrine per local protocol.

   iv. Initiate BVM ventilation as indicated (avoid intubation when able).

D. Bronchiolitis

1. Respiratory infection of the bronchioles.

2. Typically occurs in winter, in children under 2 years of age.

3. Signs and symptoms

   i. Similar to asthma

   ii. Expiratory wheezing

4. Management

   i. General management of advanced life support (ALS) patients (Patient Assessment chapter).

   ii. Place in position of comfort.

   iii. Nebulized epinephrine recommended for severe respiratory distress when oxygen and suctioning do not result in clinical improvement.

   iv. Evidence does not support use of albuterol (nebulized epinephrine recommended).

   v. Ipratropium should not be administered to pediatric patients with bronchiolitis.

   vi. IV access only necessary if dehydration is suspected or if needed for IV medications.

E. Sudden unexplained infant death (SUID) and sudden infant death syndrome (SIDS)
  1. Sudden unexplained infant death
     i. The sudden, unexpected death of an infant younger than 1 year of age.
     ii. Possible causes of SUID include suffocation, entrapment, infection, airway obstruction, cardiac dysrhythmias, trauma and SIDS.
  2. Sudden infant death syndrome
     i. Sudden death of infant from unknown etiology.
     ii. A leading cause of death in infants (especially 1–6 months old).
     iii. SIDS is one form of SUID.
  3. Management
     i. Follow normal resuscitation guidelines.
     ii. Support parents/family members.
     iii. If resuscitation is not initiated or terminated, allow family to see child.

F. Apparent life-threatening event (ALTE) and brief resolved unexplained event (BRUE)
  1. Event in infants reported by bystander as sudden and brief and completely resolved prior to EMS, including:
     i. Breathing change.
     ii. Color change.
     iii. Loss of muscle tone.
     iv. Altered LOC.
  2. ALTE/BRUE are a collection of symptoms, not a diagnosis.
  3. Transport all pediatric patients if history indicates occurrence of ALTE/BRUE.

G. Child maltreatment
  1. Forms of maltreatment
     i. Neglect
     ii. Physical abuse

- iii. Sexual abuse
- iv. Emotional abuse
- v. Other, e.g., abandonment, parental substance abuse, human trafficking

2. Perpetrators
    - i. Usually a parent or full-time caregiver.
    - ii. Often exhibit evasive or hostile behavior.
    - iii. May be experiencing crisis, financial stress, relationship issues.

3. Signs of maltreatment
    - i. Lack of supervision.
    - ii. Overly compliant, passive, or withdrawn child.
    - iii. Caregiver shows lack of concern for child.
    - iv. Unexplained injuries, fractures, burns, bruising, traumatic brain injury.
    - v. Multiple bruising in various stages of healing.
        - ➤ Red: Less than 24 hours
        - ➤ Blue/purple: 1–4 days
        - ➤ Green/yellow: 5–7 days
        - ➤ Disappearing: 1–3 weeks
    - vi. Child that shrinks at approach of adults.
    - vii. Explanations inconsistent with injury patterns.
    - viii. Signs of malnutrition.
    - ix. Frequently absent from school.
    - x. Skin infections.
    - xi. Poor hygiene/
    - xii. Delayed verbal or social skills.

4. Shaken baby syndrome/shaken impact syndrome
    - i. Form of physical abuse that occurs when the infant or child is shaken violently.
    - ii. Often happens when child won't stop crying.
    - iii. Can cause head bleeds, blindness, brain damage, skull fractures, death.

Chapter 25

5. Burns due to abuse
    i. Most burns due to abuse are from hot liquids or other hot objects.
    ii. Patterned burns (in clear shape of a hot object) and forced immersion burn patterns (stocking pattern) are indicative of abuse.
6. Management
    i. Provide proper medical attention.
    ii. Do everything possible to facilitate transport.
    iii. Report suspicions to authorities.
    iv. Document thoroughly.

H. Patients with special needs
1. Tracheostomy tube: See Airway/Oxygenation/Ventilation chapter.
2. Home ventilator
    i. 9-1-1 calls often due to mechanical failure or loss of electricity.
    ii. Switch immediately to BVM ventilation until problem resolved and transport as indicated.
3. Central line
    i. Used for long-term IV therapies.
    ii. Includes percutaneous intravenous catheter (PIC) lines.
    iii. Complications
        - Obstruction of line (clotting, cracked or kinked line)
        - Site infection
        - Hemorrhage
        - Air embolism
    iv. Management
        - Control bleeding.
        - Clamp line if large amount of air in line.
        - Place patient on left side with head down if air embolism suspected.
        - Transport.

4. Gastric tube
   i. Gastric tubes (inserted nasally into stomach) and gastronomy tubes (placed through abdominal wall into stomach) used for patients not capable of eating normally.
   ii. Complications
   - Bleeding
   - Displaced tube
   iii. Management
   - Supportive care.
   - Minimize risk of aspiration.
   - Transport.
5. Shunt
   i. Surgical procedure allowing excess cerebrospinal fluid to drain from brain to abdomen, reducing risk of increased ICP.
   ii. Signs of shunt failure
   - Altered LOC
   - Posturing
   - Pupillary changes
   iii. Management
   - General management of ALS patients (Patient Assessment chapter).
   - Rapid transport for surgical intervention.

X. JumpSTART TRIAGE (MASS CASUALTY INCIDENTS)

A. Based on START triage (see Incident Management chapter).

B. If patient appears to be a child, use JumpSTART algorithm.
   i. Don't delay triage to confirm age.
   ii. See JumpSTART algorithm.

Chapter 25

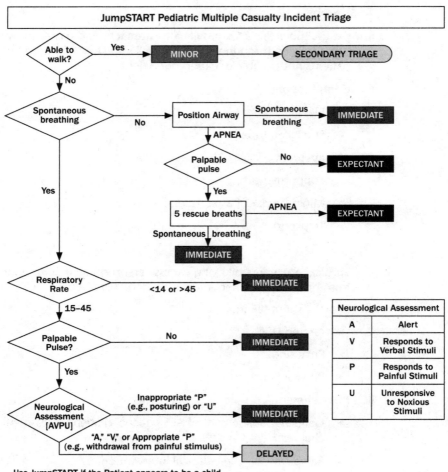

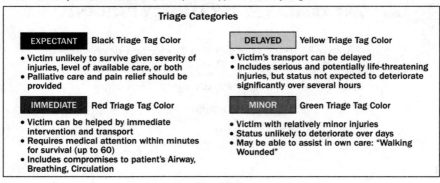

Figure 25-1.

C. JumpSTART special considerations
   i. Triage patients too young to walk and nonambulatory patients (as these patients cannot move themselves) to **green** (Minor) area.
   ii. Once **red** (Immediate) patients and **yellow** (Delayed) patients are managed, reassess **black** (Expectant) patients.

XI. CHILD PASSENGER SAFETY

A. Birth–2 years: Rear-facing seat, back seat.

B. 2–5 years: Forward-facing seat, back seat.

C. 5+ years (seatbelts fit properly): Booster seat. Belts fit properly when the lap belt lays across the upper thighs (not stomach) and the shoulder belt lays across the chest (not neck). Back seat for the best protection.

D. *Note:* Buckle all children 12 and under in back seat (middle seat preferred). Never place rear-facing seat in front of an airbag.

REVIEW QUESTIONS
(Answers on pg. 427.)

1. How long does it normally take for all of an infant's fontanelles to fully close?
   A. 3–6 months
   B. 6–12 months
   C. 12–18 months
   D. 24–36 months

Chapter 25

2. Which of the following is correct regarding management of pediatric patients?

   A. You will need to hyperextend the head to open the pediatric airway.

   B. Pediatric patients have a lower risk of head injury vs. adults.

   C. Pediatric patients are more prone to airway obstruction.

   D. A normal blood pressure in pediatric patients indicates that they are not in shock.

3. Bradycardia in pediatric patients should be regarded as a sign of _____ until proven otherwise.

   A. increased intracranial pressure

   B. cardiac tamponade

   C. hypovolemic shock

   D. hypoxia

4. Which of the following is part of the ABCs of the pediatric assessment triangle?

   A. appearance

   B. airway

   C. consciousness

   D. breath sounds (with stethoscope)

5. Based on the mother's description, you suspect that your infant patient experienced a brief resolved unexplained event (BRUE) prior to your arrival. You should:

   A. offer to transport the patient to the pediatrician's office.

   B. transport the patient to the hospital.

   C. recommend that the mother contact her child's pediatrician.

   D. report the incident as possible child abuse to the authorities.

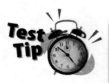

Test Tip

The national certification exam is based on the current American Heart Association (AHA) Guidelines for Basic Life Support (BLS), Advanced Cardiovascular Life Support (ACLS), and Pediatric Advanced Life Support (PALS). If you are unsure about your knowledge of these guidelines, review the appropriate AHA textbooks or equivalent publications.

Geriatrics

Chapter 26

I. TERMS TO KNOW

A. **Functional impairment:** Loss of ability to independently meet daily needs.

B. **Geriatric:** Someone who is at least 65 years of age.

C. **Polypharmacy:** Concurrent use of multiple medications.

II. AVOIDING AGEISM

A. Do not stereotype older patients.

B. Avoid use of "honey," "dear," etc.

III. PATHOPHYSIOLOGY OF AGING

A. Fragility is a better indication of the patient's well-being than age in years.

B. Leading causes of death
  1. Heart disease
  2. Cancer
  3. Stroke
  4. Respiratory conditions

Chapter 26

- C. Multisystem deterioration
  1. Physical maintenance, immune defense, and injury repair processes slow and weaken with age.
  2. Nearly 70% of elderly patients have at least two diagnosed medical conditions.
- D. Common chief complaints
  1. Weakness
  2. Dizziness, syncope
  3. Falls
  4. Headache
  5. Insomnia
  6. Loss of appetite
  7. Gastrointestinal (GI)/genitourinary problems
- E. Pharmacology
  1. Most elderly patients take at least four different prescription medications.
  2. Patients taking at least six different medications have a high risk of dangerous medication interaction.
  3. Large percentage of elderly patients do not take meds as prescribed (noncompliance).
  4. Beta-blockers
     - i. Commonly prescribed to elderly for hypertension, angina, cardiac dysrhythmias.
     - ii. Side effects often poorly tolerated in elderly.
        - ➤ Lethargy
        - ➤ Depression
        - ➤ Dizziness
        - ➤ GI problems
     - iii. Commonly prescribed beta-blockers
        - ➤ Propranolol (Inderal)
        - ➤ Atenolol

- Metoprolol
- Labetolol
5. Angiotensin-coverting enzyme (ACE) inhibitors
   i. Used for hypertension and congestive heart failure (CHF).
   ii. Commonly prescribed ACE inhibitors
      - Captopril
      - Lisinopril
      - Benazepril
   iii. Side effects
      - Hypotension
      - Vomiting
      - Diarrhea
6. Digitalis (Digoxin, Lanoxin)
   i. Widely prescribed for CHF and cardiac dysrhythmias.
   ii. Has positive inotropic and negative chronotropic effects.
   iii. High risk of toxicity, presenting with:
      - Visual disturbances.
      - Weakness, fatigue.
      - Nausea & vomiting.
      - Headache.

F. Falls
1. Elderly have a higher risk of falls than most other age groups and a higher risk of death due to fall-related injuries.

IV. GERIATRIC "GEMS DIAMOND" ASSESSMENT

A. Geriatric patients
1. Remember, geriatric patients have atypical presentations for various conditions.

Chapter 26

    B. Environmental assessment
        1. Check safety, cleanliness of patient's living environment.
        2. Working plumbing, heating, cooling, etc.
        3. Signs of alcohol abuse?
        4. Fall risks?
        5. Access to phone?
        6. Prescribed medications present and not expired?

    C. Medical assessment
        1. Expect multiple medical problems and medications.
        2. Does trauma indicate a preceding medical condition?
        3. Signs of abuse, neglect, malnutrition, dehydration, etc.

    D. Social assessment
        1. Assess activities of daily living (eating, dressing, bathing, etc.).
        2. Any difficulties obtaining food, medications, etc.
        3. Family support? Social network?

V. COMMON MEDICAL CONDITIONS IN THE ELDERLY

    A. Pneumonia
        1. Elderly pneumonia patient may not present with fever.

    B. Myocardial infarction (MI)
        1. Risk of angina, MI increases with age.
        2. Mortality rate doubles after age 70.
        3. Elderly more likely to present atypical MI symptoms.
            i. Lack of chest pain
            ii. Indigestion, epigastric pain
            iii. Dizziness, syncope
            iv. Dyspnea
            v. Fatigue

C. Congestive heart failure
   1. One of the most common cause of hospitalization after age 60.
   2. Acute myocardial infarction is a common cause of CHF.

D. Hypertension
   1. About half of all elderly patients have some degree of hypertension.
   2. Signs may be subtle in elderly.
      i. Headache
      ii. Tinnitus
      iii. Epistaxis
      iv. May indicate thyroid disease.

E. Syncope
   1. One of the most common chief complaints.
   2. Indicates need for thorough advanced life support–level assessment.
   3. Always question patients who have fallen about possible syncopal episode.

F. Stroke
   1. Increased risk of stroke and transient ischemic attack (TIA) in elderly.
   2. One-third of those with TIAs will have a stroke.

G. Seizures
   1. Common causes in elderly
      i. Alcohol withdrawal
      ii. Hypoglycemia
      iii. Tumor or cerebral hemorrhage
      iv. TBI
      v. Epilepsy
      vi. Stroke

2. Common antiseizure meds
    i. Tegretol
    ii. Zarontin
    iii. Neurontin
    iv. Keppra
    v. Luminal
    vi. Dilantin
    vii. Depakote
    viii. Depakene
    ix. lacosamide

H. Delirium, dementia, Alzheimer's disease
    1. Delirium
        i. An acute change in mentation.
        ii. Many serious causes, some reversible.
        iii. Affects mentation more than memory.
        iv. Indicates need for high-priority transport.
    2. Dementia
        i. Slow, progressive, and often irreversible deterioration in mentation.
        ii. Affects memory more than mentation.
        iii. Usually caused by Alzheimer's disease.
        iv. Does not usually require high-priority transport.
    3. Alzheimer's disease
        i. The most common cause of dementia.
        ii. Signs and symptoms
            ➤ Loss of recent memories
            ➤ Difficulty learning new things
            ➤ Mood swings, personality changes
            ➤ Wandering, often at night

- ➤ Functional impairment
- ➤ Frequent falls
- ➤ Regression to infant stage

I. Parkinson's disease
1. Degenerative disorder.
2. Signs and symptoms
    i. Tremors
    ii. Ambulatory difficulties, shuffling gait
    iii. Loss of facial expression
    iv. Muscle rigidity
    v. Jerky motion
    vi. Slow, monotone speech

J. Suicide
1. Highest suicide rates in patients (especially males) over 65.

K. Trauma and falls
1. Increased risk of injury and death, even from ground-level falls.
2. Risk factors
    i. Poor health
    ii. Polypharmacy, use of blood thinners, beta-blockers
    iii. Increased risk of abuse, neglect
    iv. Living in home environment without fall prevention measures
3. Most common fall-related fractures are to hip or pelvis, increasing risk of death.
4. Assume elderly fall victim has a hip or pelvic fracture until proven otherwise.

L. Elder abuse, neglect
1. Can occur domestically (at home) or institutionally (in a care center).

2. Risk factors
    i. Loss of independence
    ii. Living in nursing home or care facility or cared for by family member under great stress
3. Signs of abuse or neglect
    i. See Pediatrics chapter.
    ii. Signs of malnutrition
    iii. Bed sores/pressure sores
    iv. Poor hygiene or living conditions
4. Suspected abuse or neglect must be reported to appropriate authorities, as with suspected child abuse.

M. Herpes zoster (aka shingles)
1. Causes painful rash with blisters. Pain can continue after rash resolves.
2. Risk increases with age.
3. Chickenpox vaccine in childhood or a shingles vaccine as an adult can minimize risk of developing shingles.

REVIEW QUESTIONS
(Answers on pg. 427.)

1. Which of the following is the best indication of an elderly patient's well-being?

    A. fragility
    B. age
    C. medical history
    D. family support nearby

2. Most elderly patients:
    A. have significant cognitive decline.
    B. have either dementia or delirium.
    C. are on at least four medications.
    D. are depressed.

3. The "E" in the GEMS Diamond refers to:
    A. events leading to incident.
    B. environmental assessment.
    C. events indicating abuse.
    D. expected medical conditions.

4. A slow, progressive, irreversible deterioration in mentation is most likely due to:
    A. dementia.
    B. delirium.
    C. stroke.
    D. seizures.

5. What is the most common cause of dementia?
    A. alcoholism
    B. electrolyte imbalance
    C. Parkinson's disease
    D. Alzheimer's disease

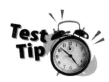

Many of the questions on the certification exam likely fall into one or both of the following categories:

1. Relates to a task that is performed frequently by paramedics.

2. Relates to a task that could harm the patient if not performed competently by the paramedic.

If it's important to know when taking care of a patient, then it's important to know before taking the certification exam.

Special Patient Populations

Chapter 27

I. TERMS TO KNOW

A. **AV shunt/fistula:** A surgical connection between an artery and vein to facilitate dialysis.

B. **Colostomy:** Surgical opening between colon and abdominal wall to allow passage of feces while bypassing part of colon.

C. **CVAD:** Central venous access device, aka central line.

D. **Cystic fibrosis:** Inherited disorder that affects lungs and digestive system.

E. **Intraventricular shunt:** Allows excess cerebrospinal fluid in brain to drain, reducing risk of increased intracranial pressure.

F. **Multiple sclerosis:** Chronic central nervous system disease in which the immune system eats away at protective covering of nerves.

G. **Muscular dystrophy:** Collection of genetic diseases that cause progressive weaknesses and degeneration of voluntary muscle.

> ➤ *Remember:* Two-thirds of domestic violence victims have injuries to the face, neck, head, or arms.

II. AT-RISK POPULATIONS

A. At-risk populations
   1. Examples: pediatrics, geriatric, economically disadvantaged, domestic violence victims, human trafficking.

365

Chapter 27

    2. Common presentation of victims of human trafficking
- i. Bruises in various stages of healing
- ii. Scars or infections
- iii. Pelvic pain, rectal trauma
- iv. Pregnancy
- v. Malnourishment
- vi. Dental problems
- vii. Phobias, panic attacks

III. PATIENTS WITH SENSORY IMPAIRMENTS

A. Hearing impaired
1. Face the patient and speak clearly.
2. Consider communicating in writing or using closed-ended questions.
3. Family members may be able to assist with communication.

B. Vision impaired
1. Communicate verbally what you are doing.
2. Keep the patient informed.
3. Protect the patient while moving.

C. Speech impaired
1. Ask questions that allow concise answers.
2. Allow the patient time to respond and do not finish the patient's statements.
3. Do not pretend you understand what the patient is saying if you do not.

Special Patient Populations

IV. DEVELOPMENTAL DISABILITIES

A. Most developmental disabilities affect the central nervous system in some way.

B. Do not assume that the patient's physical appearance is an indication of cognitive dysfunction.

C. Communicate directly with the patient and keep them informed.

D. The patient's family is typically a great resource. Listen to them.

E. Attempt to determine the patient's baseline, and what is different today.

V. PATIENTS WITH TRAUMATIC BRAIN INJURY

A. Often rely on extensive medical equipment (ventilators, infusion pumps, feeding tubes, catheters, etc.).

B. Airway and respiratory problems, urinary tract infections, and malnutrition are common.

C. Use caution when manipulating medical equipment.

VI. DIALYSIS PATIENTS

A. Patients typically have an implanted device, such as an arteriovenous (AV) shunt, fistula, or graft. These devices connect an artery and a vein to facilitate dialysis.

B. Do **not** take a blood pressure on an extremity with an AV shunt, fistula, or graft.

C. Bleeding from AV shunts or fistulas can be severe.

D. Monitor patient for bleeding, shock, or infection.

Chapter 27

- E. Dialysis patients are prone to hypotension and electrolyte imbalances (acute hypercalcemia, hypernatremia, and hypokalemia).
- F. Monitor ECG for indications of acute electrolyte emergencies.
    1. Hypokalemia
        i. T-wave may be wider, lower, flattened, or inverted.
        ii. ST-segment depression and increased PR interval.
    2. Hypercalcemia
        i. Shortened QT interval.
        ii. ST elevation.
        iii. Ventricular irritability.

VII. HOME CARE PATIENTS

- A. Pathophysiology of home care patients
    1. Most are female and 65 or older.
    2. Most informal caregivers (often family) spend at least 4 hours per day providing care, every day.
    3. Medicare funding for home care is inadequate, increasing burden on EMS system.
- B. Common EMS response for home care patients
    1. Equipment assistance or failure.
    2. Loss of caregiver.
    3. Transportation needed.
- C. Common home care medical equipment
    1. Common devices
        i. Home oxygen
        ii. Tracheostomy tubes
        iii. Home ventilators
        iv. Apnea monitors

- v. Continuous positive airway pressure or bilevel positive airway pressure machines
- vi. Small volume nebulizer machines
- vii. Surgical drains
- viii. Medication infusion pumps, analgesia pumps
- ix. Central IV catheters, "central line," central venous access device
- x. Feeding tubes
- xi. Foley catheters
- xii. Colostomy
- xiii. Peritoneal dialysis equipment
- xiv. Shunts and fistulas
- xv. Hospital-style beds
- xvi. Intraventricular shunt

2. General management
   - i. Infection, hemorrhage, and respiratory compromise are common complications with home care devices.
   - ii. Stabilize immediate airway, breathing, or circulatory problems and transport.
   - iii. See Table 27-1: Common Equipment Complications and EMS Management.

D. Special considerations
1. Attempt to determine patient's normal baseline mental status.
2. Home caregivers are often more familiar with medical equipment in the home than EMS providers.
3. Be alert for signs of abuse or neglect.
4. Home care patients can have increased risk of latex sensitivity or allergy. Have latex-free equipment options readily available.
5. Ventilator-dependent patients
   - i. For suspected malfunction: Immediately switch to bag-valve-mask (BVM) ventilation.

Table 27-1: Common Equipment Complications and EMS Management

	Common Complications	Management
Tracheostomy tube	• Mucus blockage • Dislodgement	• DOPE assessment: Displaced? Obstructed? Pneumothorax? Equipment malfunction? • Suction as indicated • Remove tube as needed • Consider inserting endotracheal tube into stoma • Initiate BVM as indicated
Home ventilator	• Ventilator malfunction • Loss of electricity	• Switch to BVM
Central vascular access devices/central line (aka Hickman, Broviac, Groshong)	• Infection • Accidental removal	• Control bleeding • Transport
Dialysis shunt	• Infection • Hemorrhage	• Do NOT apply BP cuff or start IV on same extremity • Transport
Urinary catheter	• Infection • Failure to drain	• Transport
Intraventricular shunt	• Obstruction • Increased ICP • Hypertension • Altered level of consciousness • Seizures	• Rapid transport

Special Patient Populations

  ii. For suspected respiratory acidosis/hypoxia: Increase rate and/or tidal volume.

  iii. For suspected respiratory alkalosis/hypocapnia: Decrease rate and/or tidal volume.

VIII. SPECIFIC CONDITIONS

 A. Bronchopulmonary dysplasia (BPD)
  1. Usually affects low-birth-weight infants.
  2. Often patients requires continuous mechanical ventilator support.
  3. Increased risk of respiratory infections.
  4. Pulmonary edema develops easily with excessive fluid administration.

 B. Cystic fibrosis (CF)
  1. Causes chronic and copious overproduction of mucus, airway inflammation, and infections.
  2. Most patients die before age 40.
  3. Home management often involves manual or mechanical chest percussion.
  4. Dyspnea, hemoptysis, pneumothorax, cor pulmonale are common complications.

 C. Guillain-Barre syndrome
  1. Autoimmune disorder causing muscle weakness leading to paralysis.
  2. Paralysis starts in distal extremities and moves to core, risking respiratory paralysis.
  3. Affects motor function more than sensory function.
  4. Recoverable with adequate ventilatory support.

 D. Homelessness and poverty
  1. Increased risk of poor health, mental health problems.
  2. Path from healthcare costs to bankruptcy to homelessness is common.

3. Males, Black Americans, Native Americans, LGBTQ+ youth at increased risk.

4. Advocate for patient. Connect patient to available community resources.

E. Multiple sclerosis

1. Chronic, unpredictable central nervous system (CNS)/immune disorder.

2. Immune system mistakenly attacks healthy CNS tissue.

F. Muscular dystrophy

1. Causes muscle degeneration and atrophy.

2. Patients often have difficulty ambulating.

3. Most EMS calls related to respiratory problems or fall injuries.

G. Myasthenia gravis

1. Causes weakness and fatigue of voluntary muscles.

2. Respiratory compromise possible, often preceded by difficulty swallowing or dyspnea.

REVIEW QUESTIONS
(Answers on pg. 428.)

1. Most domestic violence patients have injuries to the face, neck, head, or:
   A. legs.
   B. arms.
   C. trunk.
   D. buttocks.

Special Patient Populations

2. Which of the following is an inherited disorder that affects the lungs and digestive system?

   A. Guillain-Barre syndrome

   B. multiple sclerosis

   C. cystic fibrosis

   D. myasthenia gravis

3. Most developmental disabilities affect the:

   A. central nervous system.

   B. peripheral nervous system.

   C. immune system.

   D. endocrine system.

4. The "D" in DOPE assessment for endotracheal tube placement represents:

   A. diminished lung sounds.

   B. drop in SpO_2.

   C. displaced tube.

   D. dynamic $ETCO_2$ changes.

5. You are caring for a patient on a home ventilator. The ventilator alarm is going off and you are unsure if it is functioning properly. You should first:

   A. remove the ventilator and use a BVM.

   B. turn off the alarm.

   C. transport the patient with the ventilator.

   D. contact medical direction for assistance.

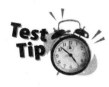

Memorizing all those flashcards you are (hopefully) making is a lot of work, but it's worth it! Treat each flashcard like it's going to earn you one more correct answer on the certification exam. Try to memorize 5–10 new flashcards each day. Set aside time every day to review the flashcards you've already memorized.

PART VIII
EMS OPERATIONS

Ground and Air Ambulance Operations

Chapter 28

I. TERMS TO KNOW

A. **Defensive driving:** Utilization of safe practices for vehicle operations in spite of surrounding conditions and the actions of others.

B. **Disinfection:** Use of a chemical to kill pathogens (there are low, medium, and high levels of disinfection).

C. **Due regard:** Emergency vehicle operators are expected to drive safely at all times and may be held to a higher standard than other drivers.

D. **System status management:** Use of data to anticipate demand for EMS services and adjust staffing levels and staging locations accordingly.

II. GROUND AMBULANCE OPERATIONS

A. Ambulance designs
   1. Type I: Truck cab-chassis with modular ambulance body.
   2. Type II: Standard van with integral cab-body ambulance.
   3. Type III: Specialty van with integral cab-body ambulance.
   4. Heavy-duty emergency vehicle.

B. Ambulance minimum standards
   1. Separate compartment for driver and patient/attendant.
   2. Room for at least two patients and attendants.
   3. Stocked with all required equipment and supplies (per state standards).

4. Radio communication with dispatchers.
5. Ability to contact medical direction.
6. Meets all federal, state, local safety standards.
7. Meets state standards for state certified ambulance.
8. Typically displays "star of life" emblem.

C. Phases of an ambulance call
1. Preparation
    i. Ambulance inspection at start of shift.
2. Dispatch
    i. Obtain essential information (location, mechanism of injury/nature of illness, etc.).
    ii. Notify dispatch you are en route.
3. Travel to scene
    i. Safe response with due regard and defensive driving habits.
    ii. Intersections are dangerous!
4. Patient contact
    i. Notify dispatch you are on scene.
    ii. Position ambulance for safe patient loading.
5. Transfer to ambulance
    i. Safely transfer and load patient in ambulance (**not** exposed to oncoming traffic).
6. Transport to receiving facility
    i. Notify dispatch you are en route.
    ii. Safe transport to appropriate receiving facility.
    iii. Intersections are dangerous!
    iv. Ensure patient(s) and attendant(s) are properly secured.
7. Transfer of care
    i. Notify dispatch you are at the hospital.
    ii. Provide verbal and written transfer of care report.

8. Return to service
    i. Decontaminate ambulance and restock as indicated (review disinfection levels, in Hematology and Infectious Disease chapter).
    ii. Notify dispatch you are back in service.

D. Due regard
    1. Emergency vehicle operators can, typically, disregard most traffic laws when responding in emergency mode.
    2. Emergency vehicle operators are required to exercise due regard at all times.
    3. Never:
        i. Never speed through a school zone.
        ii. Never pass a school bus with stop sign extended.
        iii. Never cross railroad tracks with gates down.

E. Escorts and multiple-vehicle responses
    1. Police escorts are **not** recommended unless needed for scene safety or you are lost.
    2. Exercise extreme caution with multiple-vehicle responses, especially at intersections. Likelihood of encountering another emergency vehicle increases as responding vehicles approach the scene.

> *Remember:* Safety first! Safety during emergency vehicle operations is the priority, not speed. While the attendant is responsible for patient care during transport, the emergency vehicle operator is responsible for the safety of everyone in the vehicle.

F. Defensive driving tactics
    1. Do **not** sacrifice safety for speed.
    2. Know your route.
    3. All occupants should be properly restrained during ambulance operations.
    4. All equipment should be secured (no potential projectiles).

5. Use daytime running lights.
6. Use both lights and siren when driving in emergency mode.
7. Always know what is next to you while driving.
8. Maintain safe following distance.
9. Avoid backing up whenever possible and always use a spotter.
10. Scan the road continuously.
11. Don't tunnel vision on vehicle directly in front of you.
12. Anticipate unexpected actions from other drivers.
13. Minimize distractions while driving.
14. Assume other drivers do not see or hear you.
15. Know your blind spots.
16. Pass on the left whenever possible.
17. Stop at all red lights, clear all intersections.
18. Account for ambulance's higher center of gravity and increased braking distance.
19. Exercise extreme caution in intersections, at night, and during inclement weather.
20. Do not develop lights and siren "lead foot."
21. Recognize fatigue as one of the biggest threats to safe vehicle operation.

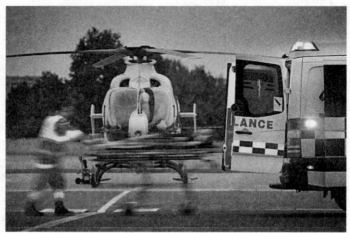

Figure 28-1: Air Ambulance.

Ground and Air Ambulance Operations

 III. AIR AMBULANCE OPERATIONS

A. Types of air ambulances

1. Rotor-wing (helicopters)

    i. Used for scene calls and local interfacility transports.

2. Fixed-wing (plane/jet)

    i. Typically for interfacility transports over 100 miles.

B. Landing zones (LZ) for rotor-wing aircraft

1. Keep LZ clear on approach and during takeoff. Aircraft may return to LZ unexpectedly and abruptly due to mechanical problems.

2. LZ should be at least 75' × 75' (day) and 100' × 100' (night) on firm, level ground and clear of overhead obstructions.

3. Ensure LZ clear of loose debris that could be caught in rotor wash.

4. Do not light LZ with caution tape, flares, unweighted lights, or blinding strobes.

5. Establish and maintain radio contact with aircraft during approach, landing, and takeoff.

C. Working around EMS helicopters

1. Never approach aircraft without the pilot's permission.

2. Never approach aircraft from the rear.

3. Secure all loose items on patient, stretcher, and EMS personnel (hats, blankets, etc.).

4. Follow local protocols regarding appropriate use of EMS helicopters and rotor-wing safety.

Chapter 28

REVIEW QUESTIONS
(Answers on pg. 429.)

1. What are ambulance operators required to do at all times while responding to an emergency?

    A. Obey speed limits.

    B. Exercise due regard.

    C. Stop at all four-way intersections.

    D. Avoid railroad crossings.

2. Emergency vehicle operators should never (select TWO):

    A. speed through a school zone.

    B. drive more than 10 miles over the posted speed limit.

    C. drive over railroad tracks.

    D. park in a fire zone.

    E. pass a school bus with its stop sign extended.

3. Which of the following are habits of defensive drivers? (Select THREE.)

    A. Always know what is next to you.

    B. Always maintain a 500' following distance.

    C. Pass on the right whenever possible.

    D. Anticipate unexpected actions from other drivers.

    E. Scan the road continuously.

    F. Focus on the vehicle directly in front of you.

4. What size is recommended for a rotor-wing landing zone at night?

    A. at least 50' × 50'

    B. at least 75' × 75'

    C. at least 100' × 100'

    D. at least 500' × 500'

Ground and Air Ambulance Operations

5. Which of the following are recommended to reduce the risk of accidents due to fatigue?

   A. Limit shift work to 48 hours or less.

   B. Allow EMS personnel to nap on duty.

   C. Encourage EMS personnel to take caffeine.

   D. Revoke driving status of those who complain of fatigue.

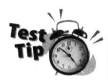

> You are likely to see fewer EMS Operations questions on the exam than the other categories; however, you still need to prepare for this topic. Make sure you are familiar with the National Incident Management System (NIMS), triage standards, and safety considerations for all types of EMS operations.

Incident Management

Chapter 29

I. TERMS TO KNOW

A. **JumpSTART:** START triage for pediatric patients.

B. **NIMS:** National Incident Management System.

C. **Primary triage:** Takes place early during incident, when patients are first encountered.

D. **Safety officer (SO):** Monitors all on-scene activities to identify and prevent harmful conditions.

E. **SALT triage:** Sort, assess, lifesaving interventions, treatment/transport.

F. **Secondary triage:** Ongoing triage completed throughout incident.

G. **Singular command:** Single individual has command of incident. Usually used for single-jurisdiction incidents.

H. **Span of control:** Number of people or tasks that one individual can manage.

I. **Staging:** Positioning of resources, such as ambulances, to allow coordinated access to scene and egress from scene with patients.

J. **START triage:** Simple triage and rapid treatment.

K. **Triage:** Sorting patients based on severity of injury.

L. **Unified command:** Multiple personnel from different jurisdictions share command.

Chapter 29

 II. NATIONAL INCIDENT MANAGEMENT SYSTEM (NIMS)

A. Purpose and origin

1. NIMS priorities are life safety, incident stabilization, and property conservation.
2. Standards set by Department of Homeland Security (DHS).
3. Comprehensive national approach to incident management. Provides adaptive, standardized approach to any type of domestic incident, e.g., terrorism or natural disaster.
4. Standardizes the command structure, terminology, and training at all jurisdictional levels and across functional disciplines.
5. Useful on full spectrum of incidents, regardless of size, location, or complexity.
6. Designed to be adaptable and flexible. Improves communication and interaction among multiple and diverse agencies at local, state, and federal levels.
7. For additional information and training about NIMS, visit:
    i. https://www.usfa.fema.gov/a-z/nims/command-and-coordination.html
    ii. www.fema.gov/emergency-managers/national-preparedness/training

B. NIMS practices

1. Coordinate efforts through a unified command or single command system to reduce duplication of effort and freelancing.
2. Use "clear text" communication to improve interagency communication and efficiency.
3. Limit span of control to no more than seven workers per supervisor.

C. Command staff

1. Incident command
    i. Incident commander responsible for overall management of the incident.
    ii. Command may be singular or unified.

Incident Management

        iii. Ideal span of control should not exceed five people or tasks (never more than seven).

        iv. Four sections under Command utilized as need to maintain span of control.

- Finance and administration
- Logistics
- Operations
- Planning

  2. Safety officer

        i. Has authority to stop any action deemed an immediate life threat.

  3. Liaison officer

        i. Coordinates incident operations involving outside agencies.

  4. Information officer

        i. Collects incident data and communicates with media.

> **Remember:** Determine if there is a designated triage method in your area. A good understanding of START triage and SALT triage will prepare you for triage-related questions on the national certification exam.

D. EMS operations

  1. Preparedness

        i. EMS agencies should have written disaster plans that should be routinely practiced and improved.

        ii. Plans should include processes to assist families of responders so responders can focus on their duties.

  2. EMS branches (under Operations)

        i. Triage

        ii. Treatment

        iii. Transportation

Chapter 29

3. Triage
    i. Purpose of triage
        - To sort patients and determine appropriate use of resources.
        - To improve patient outcomes.
    ii. Triage standards
        - Triage protocols should meet all model uniform core criteria (MUCC) identified by the National Association of EMS Physicians and the CDC, including:
            — Be easy to use.
            — Be easy to remember.
            — Should **not** rely on numbers or vitals.
        - *Note:* Regardless of the triage system being used, all patients with altered level of consciousness or signs of shock should be considered "Immediate."
    3. Primary and secondary triage
        - Primary triage: initial triage, completed upon first encounter with patient.
        - Secondary triage: ongoing triage, for example triaging again once patient arrives in the treatment area.
    iv. Triage systems
        - START and JumpSTART triage
            — START Triage (adults): See START Triage algorithm.
            — JumpSTART (pediatrics): See Pediatrics chapter.
            — Do not meet MUCC.
        - SALT triage
            — **S**ort; **A**ssess; **L**ifesaving interventions; **T**reatment/transport.
            — Meets all MUCC.

Incident Management

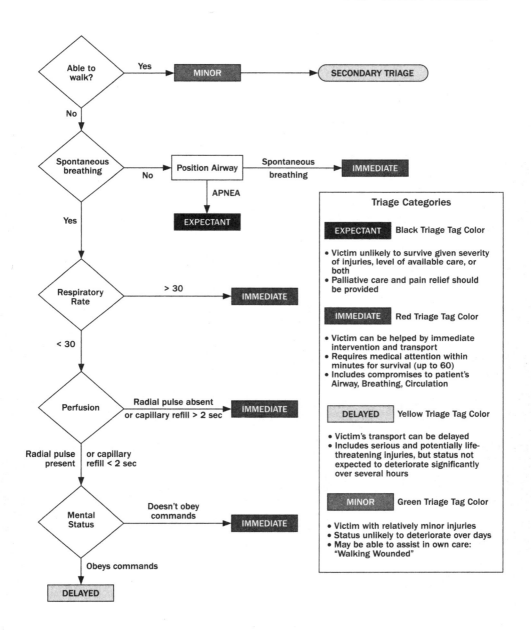

Figure 29-1: START Flowchart

Source: U.S. National Library of Medicine

Chapter 29

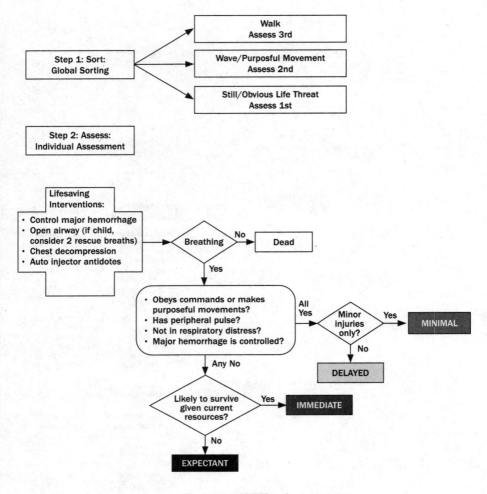

Figure 29-2: SALT Flowchart

Adapted from: SALT mass casualty triage: concept endorsed by the American College of Emergency Physicians, American College of Surgeons Committee on Trauma, American Trauma Society, National Association of EMS Physicians, National Disaster Life Support Education Consortium, and State and Territorial Injury Prevention Directors Association. Disaster Med Public Health Prep. 2008 Dec;2(4):245-6. [PubMed Citation]

III. DISASTER MENTAL HEALTH SERVICES

A. Designed to assist those experiencing critical incident stress.

B. Focuses on meeting basic human needs.

   1. Listening, compassion

2. Ensuring basic physical needs are met
3. Encouraging social support
4. Protecting from additional harm

REVIEW QUESTIONS
(Answers on pg. 429.)

1. Why does the NIMS recommend coordinating efforts through either a unified command or a single command system?
    A. to reduce incident management costs.
    B. to reduce duplication of effort.
    C. to allow incident commanders to practice their skills.
    D. to qualify for federal emergency management funding.

2. Which of the following is a recommended practice during a mass casualty, multiagency incident?
    A. Use clear text communication.
    B. Switch to law enforcement radio frequencies.
    C. Identify an incident commander from each agency.
    D. Limit span of control to no more than 10 people per supervisor.

3. During a mass casualty incident, who has the authority to stop any action deemed a life threat?
    A. the triage officer
    B. the highest-ranking paramedic
    C. the information officer
    D. the safety officer

4. According to NIMS, triage, treatment, and transportation fall under the:
    A. operations section.
    B. planning section.
    C. logistics section.
    D. administrative section.

Chapter 29

5. The purpose of triage is to:

   A. immediately stabilize life-threatening conditions.

   B. determine the best use of limited resources.

   C. identify all Level 1 trauma patients quickly.

   D. limit the response of unnecessary resources.

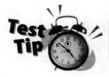

Safety First! You are likely to see several safety-related questions on the certification exam. An answer choice related to your safety is usually the correct response.

Rescue Operations, Hazardous Materials, Terrorism

Chapter 30

I. TERMS TO KNOW

A. **Biotoxin:** Poisonous substance produced by living organism, such as ricin and botulinum toxin.

B. **CBRNE:** Chemical, biological, radiological, nuclear, explosives.

C. **Complex access:** Requires use of special tools and training to access/extricate patient.

D. **Cribbing:** Using timber to temporarily support weight of an unstable object during rescue operations, such as a vehicle on its roof.

E. **Dirty bomb:** A nuclear weapon improvised from radioactive nuclear waste material and conventional explosives.

F. **Emergency move:** Used when dangers require immediate movement of the patient.

G. **Entrapment:** Being trapped in an enclosed space.

H. **Extrication:** Removal of a patient from entrapment.

I. **Incapacitating agents:** Used for riot control or personal protection, such as mace and pepper spray.

J. **Incendiary agents:** Explosives with less power but greater heat and burn potential, such as napalm.

K. **Pulmonary agents:** Chemical agents that damage the lungs, such as phosgene, chlorine, and hydrogen sulfide.

Chapter 30

    L. **Safety data sheet (SDS):** Contain detailed information about all hazardous substances on site (formerly called material safety data sheets (MSDS).

    M. **Shoring:** Provides temporary support of damaged or collapsed structure to conduct search and rescue operations.

    N. **Simple access:** Gaining access to the patient without tools or breaking glass.

    O. **Urgent move:** Used when patient has potential life threats and must be moved quickly.

    P. **Vesicant:** Blistering chemical agent, such as mustard gas, lewisite, and phosgene oxime.

II. EMS ROLE DURING SPECIAL OPERATIONS

    A. Many incidents require personnel with specialized training. Do not attempt operations you have not been trained for.

    B. EMS providers' primary role is personal safety and patient care once it is safe to do so.

    C. Always wear personal protective equipment (PPE) appropriate for the situation.

    D. Special operations may include:
       1. Vehicle extrication.
       2. Search and rescue/technical rescue.
       3. Water rescue.
       4. Structure fire.
       5. Law enforcement operations.
       6. Hazmat incidents.
       7. Natural disasters.
       8. Mass casualty incidents.

III. EXTRICATION OPERATIONS

A. Scene safety

1. Leather gloves should be worn over (not instead of) regular PPE gloves when working around glass, sharp objects, rope, etc.
2. Federal law requires use of an approved, highly reflective traffic safety vest when working on roadways, near traffic, or at an accident scene.
3. Review difference between cribbing and shoring (see Terms to Know).

B. Vehicle safety systems

1. Shock-absorbing bumpers
    i. Assume all modern vehicles are equipped with shock-absorbing bumpers, front and rear.
    ii. Compressed bumpers can spontaneously release with great force.
    iii. Approach damaged vehicle from sides, not front or rear.
    iv. Do **not** conduct patient care in front of or behind a damaged vehicle.
2. Supplemental restraint systems (SRS)
    i. Assume all modern vehicles are equipped with multiple SRS airbags (up to 10 is not uncommon).
    ii. Airbags deploy at about 200 mph and could be triggered accidentally following an accident (even after battery disconnected).
    iii. Maintain safe distance between you and undeployed airbags.
        ➤ Driver front airbag: at least 10".
        ➤ Knee airbag: at least 20".
        ➤ Side curtain airbag: at least 5".

C. Phases of extrication

1. Arrival and scene size-up
    i. Position vehicle to improve scene safety.

ii. Perform 360-degree walkaround if able.

iii. Determine scene hazards, number of patients, additional resources needed.

> *Remember:* All orange cables on an electric vehicle are high-voltage; however, **not all** high-voltage cables are orange.

2. Control of hazards
   i. Traffic, fuel leaks, etc.
   ii. Electric and hybrid vehicles: Do not attempt to disconnect car battery unless trained to do so.
3. Patient access
   i. Do not attempt to gain access without proper training.
   ii. Keep patient safe while rescuers conduct extrication operations, e.g., blanket, eye protection.
   iii. Rapid extrication is indicated for patients with potentially life-threatening injuries.
4. Patient care
   i. Patient care can be performed during extrication operations if safe to do so.
5. Disentanglement
   i. Simple or complex access (do not attempt complex access without proper training and equipment).
   ii. Perform emergency move or urgent move as indicated.
6. Patient packaging
   i. Complete or repeat primary assessment.
   ii. Manage immediate life threats.
   iii. Determine transport priority.
   iv. Complete thorough patient assessment (while en route if indicated).
7. Transport

IV. HAZARDOUS MATERIALS

A. Hazardous materials training

1. Awareness: Trains responders to recognize potential hazards. Federal law requires all rescue personnel to receive Awareness-level training (additional info: *https://training.fema.gov*).

2. Operations: Trains first responders to protect people, property, and the environment. Trained in use of specialized PPE.

3. Technician: Provides significant training related to halting release or spread of hazardous materials.

4. Specialist: Highest level of training. Typically provides assistance at command level.

B. Scene safety considerations

1. Hazardous materials come in many forms. Utilize all your senses to stay alert. When in doubt, get out!

2. All EMS providers should have at least Awareness-level hazmat training (*https://training.fema.gov*).

3. EMS personnel tasks on a hazmat scene include personal safety, notification of appropriate authorities, safety of the public, and patient care in a safe zone.

C. Hazmat resources

1. Emergency Response Guidebook (ERG)

2. Shipping papers

3. Safety data sheets

4. Local hazmat teams

5. CAMEO database (*https://www.epa.gov/cameo*)

6. Poison control centers/toxicologists (1-800-222-1222 or *www.poisoncontrol.org*)

D. Placards

1. Transport of hazardous materials

    i. Vehicles containing hazardous materials in certain quantities are required to display diamond-shaped identification placards.

Chapter 30

➤ Placards contain a four-digit United Nations (UN) identification number.

➤ All UN numbers listed in ERG.

➤ Report placard information when requesting additional resources if safe to do so.

ii. Drivers transporting hazardous materials are required to have shipping papers that identify the substance(s) and quantities being shipped.

iii. *Note:* Always be alert for hazardous materials in non-placarded vehicles (pool cleaners, exterminators, etc.).

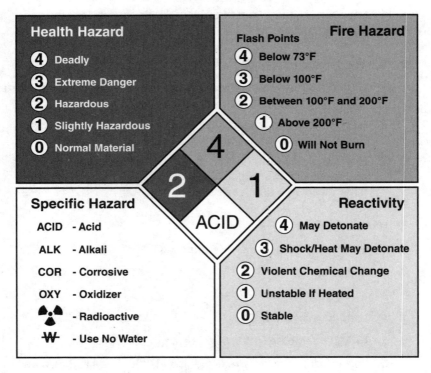

2. Fixed storage locations

   i. Diamond placards used for fixed storage locations with hazardous materials. Placard contains four smaller placards within.

   ➤ Blue diamond: Provides information about health hazards (numbered 0–4).

- Red diamond: Provides information about fire hazard (numbered 0–4).
- Yellow diamond: Provides information about reactivity hazards (numbered 0–4).
- White diamond: Displays symbols indicating special hazards (radioactivity, reactive to water, etc.).
- Numbering: The higher the number, the greater the hazard.

E. Hazmat zones
  1. Hot zone
     i. Contaminated area, requires appropriate PPE.
     ii. Those without proper training and PPE are **not** permitted in hot zone.
     iii. Patient care does **not** take place in the hot zone.
  2. Warm zone
     i. Between hot and cold zones.
     ii. Appropriate PPE required.
     iii. Only life-threatening conditions are treated in warm zone.
     iv. Everyone in warm zone must be decontaminated in warm zone before entering cold zone.
  3. Cold zone
     i. Most treatment performed in cold zone.
     ii. Typically, EMS providers remain in cold zone.

F. Decontamination
  1. Essential to prevent spread of hazardous material.
  2. Includes patient's hair, body, clothes, and any medical equipment.
  3. Decon should be performed by personnel trained and equipped to do so.

> *Remember:* To learn more about the EMS aspects of terrorism response and weapons of mass destruction, visit *https://training.fema.gov*. Look for the following online classes: Intro to ICS, Intro to NIMS, Active Shooter, Intro to Hazmat.

V. TERRORISM AND WEAPONS OF MASS DESTRUCTION (WMD)

A. Safety considerations

1. Your safety is **always** the first priority.
2. Be alert for chemical, biological, radiological, nuclear, explosive (CBRNE) hazards.
3. Follow local protocols and incident command system (ICS).

B. Chemical agents

1. Nerve agents
    i. A significant threat due to relative ease of acquisition and deployment.
    ii. Cause excessive (potentially fatal) overstimulation of the sympathetic nervous system.
    iii. Readily available organophosphates (pesticides) can be used as nerve agents.
    iv. Common organophosphate nerve agents include Sarin, Soman, Tabun, VX.
    v. Signs and symptoms (SLUDGEM/DUMBELS) and management of nerve agent exposure: See Toxicology chapter.

2. Vesicants (blistering agent)
    i. Examples: lewisite, sulfur, mustard.
    ii. Causes pain, burns, and blisters to skin, eyes, and respiratory tract.
    iii. Onset can be immediate, or delayed several hours.
    iv. Affected areas should be irrigated with copious amounts of water ASAP.

3. Cyanide (blood agent)
    i. Signs, symptoms, and management: See Toxicology chapter.

4. Pulmonary (choking) agents
    i. Examples: chlorine gas, phosgene.
    ii. Causes dyspnea, cough, wheezing, sore throat, airway irritation, and pulmonary edema.

iii. Manage ABCs (Airway, Breathing, Circulation), administer oxygen, ventilate as indicated, consider bronchodilator meds.

C. Biological agents
1. Used to cause disease.
2. Examples: anthrax, pneumonic plague, tularemia, smallpox.
3. Can cause fever, weakness, flu-like symptoms, respiratory distress.
4. Supportive care.

D. Radiological/nuclear weapons
1. Can cause injury and death from the blast, radiation, and thermal burns.
2. Radiation types
    i. Alpha radiation: Slow-moving radiation that can only travel short distances. Minimal risk due to external exposure, stopped by clothing, skin, etc. Dangerous if inhaled or ingested.
    ii. Beta radiation: Can only travel a few feet. Penetrates only the first few millimeters of skin. Serious risk if ingested or inhaled.
    iii. Gamma radiation (X-ray): Can travel long distances. Easily penetrates the body. A significant threat to living organisms (all forms of exposure).
3. Radiation sickness
    i. Nausea, vomiting
    ii. Diarrhea
    iii. Headache
    iv. Skin lesions
4. Protection
    i. **Time:** Spend as little time as possible near a radiation source.
    ii. **Distance:** Get as far away as possible from the radiation source.
    iii. **Shielding:** Gamma radiation requires extensive shielding, such as lead or concrete.

E. Explosives
   1. Most commonly used WMD.
   2. Expect significant blunt and penetrating trauma, burns, and crush injuries.
      i. Primary blast injuries: Injuries caused directly by the blast/pressure wave.
      ii. Secondary blast injuries: Injuries caused by shrapnel and flying debris.
      iii. Tertiary blast injuries: Injuries caused by striking the ground or other objects.
      iv. Quaternary: All other explosive-related injuries or disease.

F. Incapacitating agents
   1. Agents intentionally designed to incapacitate without permanent injury.
   2. Often used by law enforcement or for personal protection; however, could also be used by terrorists.
   3. Signs and symptoms
      i. Eye irritation, lacrimation (excessive tearing)
      ii. Rhinorrhea (runny nose)
      iii. Airway irritation, dyspnea
   4. Management
      i. Ensure scene safety, appropriate PPE.
      ii. Remove from source.
      iii. Remove any contaminated clothing.
      iv. Administer oxygen as indicated.
      v. Irrigation as indicated.
         ➤ Irrigate the eyes and skin as indicated for 10–20 minutes.
         ➤ Remove contact lenses.
         ➤ Use water or normal saline solution.
         ➤ Do not pour over forehead (can contaminate eyes).
         ➤ Do not force eyes open.
         ➤ Once eyes treated, have patient close eyes and irrigate entire head to prevent secondary contamination of eyes.

VI. TACTICAL EMERGENCY CASUALTY CARE (TECC)

A. TECC utilizes evidence and best practices to guide medical response and treatment during high-risk and atypical civilian operational scenarios. For additional information, visit *www.c-tecc.org*.

B. TECC phases

1. **Direct threat care:** Emphasis on mitigating the threat, moving the wounded, and managing massive hemorrhage.

2. **Indirect threat care:** Initiated once casualties are in an area of relative safety. Focus is on treating preventable causes of death.

3. **Evacuation care:** Focus is on moving casualties to definitive care, reassessing interventions, and hypothermia management.

C. EMS response to civil unrest

1. Examples of civil unrest events

    i. Periods of social upheaval

    ii. Following sporting events

    iii. Periods of extreme community tension

2. Recommendations

    i. Wear civilian clothes when reporting to or returning from duty.

    ii. Wear ballistic protection if available.

    iii. Establish a family communication plan.

    iv. Fire and EMS personnel do not participate in crowd control operations.

    v. Work in pairs or teams.

    vi. Carry a radio and flashlight.

    vii. Secure equipment (do not display scissors, etc.).

    viii. Do not wear badges.

    ix. Minimize carried equipment.

Chapter 30

> **Remember:** Know the following before taking the national certification exam:
>
> CBRNE: Types of weapons of mass destruction.
>
> SLUDGEM/DUMBELS: Nerve agent exposure signs.
>
> The three protections from radiation.
>
> The four types of blast injuries.

REVIEW QUESTIONS
(Answers on pg. 430.)

1. Using timber to temporarily support the weight of an unstable object during rescue operations is known as:

   A. shoring.

   B. cribbing.

   C. framing.

   D. loading.

2. Chemical agents that damage the lungs, such as phosgene or chlorine, are known as:

   A. pulmonary agents.

   B. incendiary agents.

   C. biotoxins.

   D. vesicants.

3. What should be worn over regular PPE gloves when working around glass, sharp objects, or rope?

   A. a second layer of PPE gloves

   B. nylon gloves

   C. static-resistant gloves

   D. leather gloves

Rescue Operations, Hazardous Materials, Terrorism

4. What is the minimum safe distance between you and an undeployed driver's front airbag?

   A. at least 5 inches

   B. at least 10 inches

   C. at least 20 inches

   D. at least 4 feet

5. You arrive on scene of a reported person down. You note a diamond placard on the entrance to the scene. The blue diamond has the number 4 on it. Blue refers to _____ hazards and the 4 indicates _____.

   A. specific hazard; slightly hazardous.

   B. instability; may detonate.

   C. health; deadly hazard.

   D. fire hazard; flash point below 73°F.

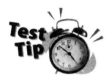

If you would like to learn more about the EMS aspects of terrorism response and WMD, visit *https://training.fema.gov/* and complete the free online IS-100.C: Introduction to Incident Command System. Here are two additional recommended courses through *www.teex.org*:

AWR111: Basic Emergency Medical Services (EMS) Concepts for Chemical, Biological, Radiological, Nuclear, and Explosive (CBRNE) Events.

AWR160: WMD/Terrorism Awareness for Emergency Responders

You Passed! Now What?

There are about 126,500 nationally certified paramedics in the U.S. That's 0.0004% of the population. Your passing score means you have accomplished something very few people ever will. Congratulations! Now what? Here are a few suggestions:

ACTION #1: CELEBRATE

You know better than most that NREMT only grants certification to those that have earned it. You have demonstrated that you have the knowledge and skills necessary to function competently as a paramedic. This accomplishment should be celebrated. Take a trip, throw a party, or just relax and decompress. Give yourself a break from the rigors of class, homework, tests, etc.

ACTION #2: EXPRESS GRATITUDE

Thank those that helped you get here, especially your family that put up with you as a tired, stressed-out paramedic student. Let your instructor know you passed. Thank anyone that made this journey a little easier for you. You will likely lean on some of these people again when you decide what your next big challenge will be.

ACTION #3: OBTAIN YOUR STATE LICENSE

In most cases, you are not employable as a paramedic until you obtain your state license. The process varies from state to state but is usually quite simple compared to what you have already accomplished. You have most likely already received instructions from your paramedic instructor. If not, contact your state EMS authority and ask them how to proceed.

ACTION #4: UPDATE YOUR RESUME

You have a lot of things to add to your resume. There are many good resume templates available. Consider asking your paramedic instructor to review your updated resume.

ACTION #5: JOIN AND READ

EMS is a dynamic profession. The one thing you can count on to stay the same is change. Much of what you learned in paramedic school will be outdated in time. Find a way to stay engaged. Consider joining the National Association of EMTs. Subscribe to one of the EMS trade journals. The two most widely recognized periodical publications in the EMS profession are the *Journal of Emergency Medical Services (JEMS)* and *EMS World*. Both publications include clinical articles, continuing education opportunities, and information about upcoming conferences.

ACTION #6: ATTEND AN EMS CONFERENCE

Research the availability of local EMS conferences in your area. This is a great way to earn continuing education credits, learn about new equipment, and network with other EMS professionals, vendors, and employers. There are some excellent national EMS conferences, such as the JEMS Conference and Expo and the EMS World Expo.

You Passed! Now What

ACTION #7: BEGIN THE RECERTIFICATION PROCESS

About the time you pass the national certification exam, it's time to start thinking about recertification. You likely have several certifications/licenses now, all with different expiration dates. You have two years before your national certification expires; however, the requirements can be extensive. Don't procrastinate. Visit the NREMT website and become familiar with the recertification process. NREMT provides some very helpful online resources to help track your recertification process. Trust me, it's much easier and less stressful to maintain your credentials than it is to get them back if they expire.

ACTION #8: DIG DEEPER

You are at the beginning – not the end – of the learning process as a paramedic. The nice thing is that now you can pick what you would like to learn more about. There are a number of additional credentials available to you. You could pursue additional training in trauma, tactical EMS, pediatrics, newborns, medical emergencies, National Incident Management System, hazardous materials, critical care, and much more. Consider doing some teaching for your local EMT program to pass on your knowledge. It's a great way to keep your skills sharp, too.

Most importantly … Stay safe, stay healthy, and continue to be a role model for your community and your profession.

Answers to Review Questions

ANATOMY & PHYSIOLOGY REVIEW CHAPTER
(See A&P review questions online at *www.rea.com/paramedic.*)

1. **A.**

    The alveoli diffuse oxygen from the respiratory system to the pulmonary capillaries in the circulatory system.

2. **C.**

    SVR is determined primarily by cardiac output and the size of arterial vessels. Vasoconstriction increases SVR and vasodilation decreases SVR.

3. **C.**

    The two divisions of the peripheral nervous system are the somatic (voluntary) and autonomic (involuntary).

4. **A., D., E.**

    Solid organs include the liver, spleen, kidneys, pancreas.

5. **B.**

    Essential functions, such as breathing, are controlled by the brain stem (midbrain, pons, medulla).

CHAPTER 1

1. **A.**

    Schedule I controlled substances (e.g., heroin, LSD) have a high potential for abuse and no accepted medical uses.

Appendix

2. **A., C., D.**

    Protocols, certification level, and cross-checks are not among the "rights" of drug administration.

3. **C.**

    $(10 \times 0.5) \div 1 = 5$

4. **B.**

    $165 \div 2.2 = 75$

5. **D.**

    The drop factor for microdrip tubing is 60 drops per mL. Macrodrip (blood) tubing has a drop factor of 10 drops per mL.

CHAPTER 2

1. **B.**

    Epinephrine is an alpha 1, beta 1, and beta 2 stimulant.

2. **A.**

    Ondansetron (Zofran) is an antiemetic.

3. **D.**

    IV dextrose can cause tissue necrosis with IV infiltration.

4. **C.**

    Diazepam (Valium) is indicated for generalized seizures.

5. **A.**

    Common side effects of fentanyl administration include CNS depression, hypotension, and nausea & vomiting.

Answers to Review Questions

CHAPTER 3

1. **A.**

   Early indications of hypoxia include restlessness, anxiousness, tachycardia, and tachypnea. Late signs include severe distress, decreased LOC, bradycardia, and cyanosis.

2. **C.**

   A normal pH is 7.35–7.45. Below 7.35 indicates acidosis, above 7.45 indicates alkalosis. Hypoxia can't be determined by the pH alone.

3. **C.**

   Inserting an ETT too far into the trachea will likely result in a right mainstem intubation.

4. **D.**

   Respiratory and cardiac arrest are contraindications for RSI. The other choices are possible indications for RSI.

5. **C., D.**

   Indications of a difficult intubation include hypersecretions, obesity, pulmonary edema, airway burns, and facial trauma.

CHAPTER 4

1. **D.**

   After the scene size-up, the primary assessment precedes all other components of patient assessment.

2. **B.**

   The purpose of the primary assessment is to identify and manage life-threatening conditions.

Appendix

3. **A.**

   Patients who are unresponsive or have life-threatening external bleeding should be assessed using the "CAB" approach.

4. **D.**

   Unresponsive patients with a pulse of 60 or below require CPR.

5. **A.**

   JVD should be assessed while the patient's head is elevated about 45 degrees. JVD is often a normal finding in supine patients.

CHAPTER 5

1. **A.**

   Leads I, II, and III are bipolar leads. aVR, aVL, and aVF are unipolar/augmented leads. V_1–V_6 are chest/precordial leads.

2. **C.**

   Inferior leads: II, III, aVF; **Septal leads:** V_1, V_2; **Anterior leads:** V_3, V_4; **Lateral leads:** I, aVL, V_5, V_6

3. **A.**

   Target ventilations to an SpO_2 of at least 95% and an $ETCO_2$ of 40 mmHg.

4. **C.**

   A normal nonfasting blood glucose level is 70–120 mg/dL. A normal fasting level is 99 mg/dL or less. A level over 200 mg/dL indicates possible diabetes.

5. **D.**

   A high SpHb indicates hemoconcentration due to low plasma (dehydration). A low SpHb indicates possible hemorrhage or anemia.

ns to Review Questions

CHAPTER 6

1. A., D., E.

   Distributive ("warm") shock includes septic, anaphylactic, and neurogenic shock. Tension pneumothorax and cardiac tamponade are examples of obstructive shock.

2. C.

   Dark stool is called melena. Hematochezia is bloody stool.

3. A.

   External bleeding is the most preventable cause of traumatic death.

4. A., C., F.

   The three primary causes of shock are pump (heart) damage, fluid loss, and vasodilation. This is known as the Perfusion Triangle.

5. D.

   A falling BP or hypotension are the best indicators of decompensated shock.

CHAPTER 7

1. A.

   Afterload is the resistance (pressure) the heart overcomes during ventricular contraction. Preload is the volume of blood returning to the heart.

2. C.

   The SA node is the primary pacemaker site. The AV node/junction is the backup.

3. B., D., E.

   ACS includes unstable angina, STEMI, and NSTEMI.

Appendix

4. C., D., F.

    Consider right ventricular infarct, PE, and cardiac tamponade for any patient with these three findings. Left heart failure and tension pneumothorax will not likely present with clear lungs. Hypovolemic shock will not likely present with JVD.

5. A., B., D.

    Left heart failure: pulmonary edema and dyspnea are common. Right heart failure: JVD and pedal edema are common.

CHAPTER 8

1. D.

    Hematemesis is vomiting blood. Epistaxis is a nosebleed.

2. A.

    External respiration is the movement of O_2 and CO_2 between the alveoli and the circulatory system. Spontaneous breathing and PPV do not ensure internal respiration.

3. B.

    Normal adult Vt is about 500 mL.

4. B.

    Oxygen should be administered as needed to maintain an SpO_2 of 95% or higher.

5. C.

    The presentation is most consistent with spontaneous pneumothorax.

Answers to Review Questions

CHAPTER 9

1. **D.**

   Inability to flex the head forward is nuchal rigidity. It is a common finding with meningitis.

2. **A.**

   The cerebrum is the largest part of the brain.

3. **A.**

   The outermost layer of the meninges is the dura mater.

4. **B., C.**

   The "A" in AEIOUTIPS stands for acidosis and alcohol.

5. **B.**

   The patient's GCS is a 6.

CHAPTER 10

1. **B.**

   Deep, rapid respirations (Kussmaul) and decreased LOC in a diabetic patient are indicative of DKA.

2. **A.**

   The adrenal glands stimulate the fight or flight response (think "adrenaline").

3. **D.**

   Insulin shock has a rapid onset. Hyperglycemic conditions have a slower onset.

4. **C.**

   This patient's presentation is consistent with pancreatitis.

5. **A.**

   Cushing's syndrome is an adrenal disorder caused by hyperadrenalism.

CHAPTER 11

1. **B.**

   Anaphylactic shock (anaphylaxis) is typically caused by circulatory collapse (massive systemic vasodilation) and respiratory failure.

2. **D.**

   Insects, plants, foods, medications, and radiographic contrast media are all common causes of anaphylaxis.

3. **C.**

   Epinephrine must be administered rapidly to reverse the effects of anaphylactic shock.

4. **A.**

   Glucagon may be effective for anaphylaxis patients on beta-blockers who are unresponsive to epinephrine.

5. **B.**

   Nausea, vomiting, and diarrhea are most common in food-induced anaphylaxis.

CHAPTER 12

1. **B.**

   Bruising around the umbilicus (Cullen's sign) may indicate internal hemorrhage or pancreatitis.

Answers to Review Questions

2. D.

Esophageal varices is usually due to cirrhosis secondary to alcohol abuse.

3. C.

The patient's age, sex, history, and history of present illness (HPI) are most consistent with peptic ulcer.

4. A.

The patient's age and HPI are most consistent with ulcerative colitis.

5. B.

The patient's presentation is most consistent with appendicitis.

CHAPTER 13

1. A.

Signs of symptoms of anticholinergic poisoning: "hot as Hades," "blind as a bat," "dry as a bone," "red as a beet," "mad as a hatter."

2. C.

Cholinergics/organophosphates present with "DUMBELS" or "SLUDGEM."

3. D.

Patients with cholinergic poisoning, such as pesticides or nerve agents, require high doses of atropine (2–5 mg).

4. D.

Activated charcoal is contraindicated for acid or alkali ingestion.

5. B.

The patient is presenting with signs and symptoms of a hallucinogenic overdose.

Appendix

CHAPTER 14

1. A.

Sickle cell disease is an inherited form of anemia and primarily affects people of African, Mediterranean, and Middle Eastern descent.

2. B., E.

Covid-19, influenza, and varicella are viruses and will not respond to antibiotic treatment.

3. C.

Hepatitis B is a highly infectious blood-borne pathogen.

4. D.

Respiratory syncytial virus (RSV) is highly infectious and requires an N95, KN95, or HEPA mask.

5. D.

These signs and symptoms are consistent with laryngotracheobronchitis (croup).

CHAPTER 15

1. B., C., E.

Not all patients with mental illness are violent. Unresponsive patients are not likely to be violent. Elderly patients are not more likely to be violent.

2. C.

Open-ended questions are recommended. These calls take time. Do not use ultimatums or yell.

3. D.

Dementia has a slow onset and includes conditions such as Alzheimer's disease and Parkinson's disease.

Answers to Review Questions

4. **A.**

   Excessive fasting is anorexia. Recurrent episodes of binge eating followed by self-induced vomiting or diarrhea is bulimia.

5. **C.**

   The national Suicide and Crisis Lifeline is 988.

CHAPTER 16

1. **B.**

   Conjunctivitis is also known as "pink eye."

2. **D.**

   Do not remove impaled objects from the eye. Stabilize the object and close both eyes.

3. **A.**

   Patients with a nosebleed are at increased risk for nausea and vomiting.

4. **C.**

   Ludwig's angina (inflammation under the tongue) can develop rapidly and cause airway obstruction.

5. **B.**

   Chemical burns to the eyes should be continuously irrigated with sterile saline.

CHAPTER 17

1. **A.**

   Rheumatoid arthritis is an autoimmune disease affecting joints and surrounding tissue.

2. **B.**

   The patient's presentation is most consistent with gout.

3. **D.**

   Fibromyalgia causes widespread pain in muscles and is often associated with fatigue, anxiety, or depression.

4. **B.**

   Osteoarthritis is the most common cause of chronic disability in older adults.

5. **A.**

   Osteoporosis is the most common form of bone disease. Osteoarthritis affects the joints.

CHAPTER 18

1. **A., D., F.**

   Time of injury, severity of pain, and last tetanus shot are all part of the wound history.

2. **A.**

   The radial pulse should be used to assess pulses distal to the ulna.

3. **B.**

   There is an increased risk of crush syndrome if an extremity has been trapped for a prolonged period.

4. **A., B.**

   Pulse rate over 110 (in adults) and respiratory rate over 12 (adults) are indications for transport after a taser incident.

5. **C.**

   Apply an occlusive dressing to reduce the risk of air embolism.

Answers to Review Questions

CHAPTER 19

1. D.

   About 60% of thermal burns involve children aged 5 or under.

2. A., C., D.

   Systemic complications of burn injuries include infection, hypothermia, hypovolemia, organ failure, and respiratory compromise.

3. C.

   Zone of coagulation: center of burn. Zone of stasis: adjacent to zone of coagulation, with inflammation and decreased perfusion. Zone of hyperemia: outermost area with the least damage.

4. A., E., F.

   The best protections from radiation injury are time, distance, and shielding.

5. D.

   Critical burn patients should have two large-bore IVs with lactated Ringer's (preferred over normal saline).

CHAPTER 20

1. B., D., F.

   Cushing's response (triad) indicates increased ICP and includes hypertension, bradycardia, and abnormal respirations.

2. B.

   The cerebrum is the largest portion of the brain and performs many higher cognitive functions.

423

3. A.

Epidural hematomas are usually arterial bleeds that cause a rapid increase in intracranial pressure, rapid decrease in cerebral perfusion pressure, and an acute loss of consciousness.

4. C.

Anisocoria (unequal pupils) may be an indication of increased intracranial pressure.

5. B., D., E.

Management of TBI should include preventing hypoxia, hypotension, and hyperventilation.

CHAPTER 21

1. C.

Grey Turner's sign (bruising of the flanks) may indicate retroperitoneal bleeding, ruptured ectopic pregnancy, or acute pancreatitis.

2. C.

Abnormal JVD may indicate cardiac tamponade, tension pneumothorax, pulmonary embolism, or right heart failure.

3. A.

Fractures to ribs 1–3 and 9–12 indicate a high likelihood of significant internal injuries.

4. C.

Patients with a flail chest and inadequate breathing must be ventilated immediately.

5. A.

Patients with a tension pneumothorax will typically present with dyspnea, diminished or absent lung sounds on the affected side, and hypotension (hemodynamic compromise). Tracheal deviation is a very late sign and should not be relied on as an indicator of tension pneumothorax.

Answers to Review Questions

CHAPTER 22

1. **C.**

   Age, health, and medications are all predisposing risk factors for heat and cold emergencies.

2. **A.**

   Heat exhaustion is a mild to moderate heat-related emergency caused by dehydration and electrolyte imbalance.

3. **B.**

   Severe hypothermia is the most likely environmental condition to present with decreased LOC, bradycardia, bradypnea, and new-onset a-fib.

4. **C.**

   Management of hypothermic patients with a core temperature below 86°F includes:

   - One shock only for VF.
   - Continue CPR.
   - Withhold medications.

   Follow standard ACLS guidelines for patients with a core temperature above 86°F.

5. **D.**

   CPR is indicated for unresponsive pediatric patients with a pulse below 60.

CHAPTER 23

1. **A.**

   GTPAL includes gravida, term births, preterm births, abortions, and living children.

425

Appendix

2. **A.**

   Harvard T.H. Chan School of Public Health identified homicide as the leading cause of death, over obstetric complications.

3. **C.**

   To prevent supine hypotensive syndrome, tilt the mother to her left side between 15 and 30 degrees.

4. **A.**

   Indications that delivery is imminent include crowning and the urge to push.

5. **C.**

   You should suspect placenta previa for a woman with painless vaginal bleeding in the third trimester of pregnancy.

CHAPTER 24

1. **A.**

   About 10% of newborns require assistance to start breathing. About 1% require full resuscitative measures.

2. **B.**

   These findings in a newborn are consistent with a diaphragmatic hernia.

3. **A.**

   The first action is to provide ventilations. If the heart rate remains below 60 after ventilations, then begin chest compressions.

4. **D.**

   The correction compression to ventilation ratio for newborn CPR is 3:1.

5. **C.**

   Routine use of a bulb syringe in newborns is not recommended. Dextrose 10% is recommended for a blood glucose below 45 mg/dL.

Answers to Review Questions

...are recommended if the pulse is 60 or below after Chest compressions...
providin...

CHAPTER 25

1. C.

The posterior fontanelle closes within the first couple months. The anterior fontanelle closes by 18 months.

2. C.

Pediatric patients have a larger tongue in proportion to their airway, so airway obstruction is more likely. Pediatric patients have a larger head in proportion to their body, and have an increased risk of head injuries. You should **NOT** hyperextend the pediatric patient's airway. Hypotension is a **late** sign of shock.

3. D.

Bradycardia should be regarded as a sign of hypoxia in pediatric patients until proven otherwise.

4. A.

The ABCs of the PAT: <u>A</u>ppearance, work of <u>B</u>reathing, <u>C</u>irculation to skin.

5. B.

Infants that appear to have experienced an apparent life-threatening event (ALTE) or brief resolved unexplained event (BRUE) should be transported to the hospital for physician evaluation.

CHAPTER 26

1. A.

The patient's fragility is the best of the four indicators of an elderly patient's well-being.

Appendix

2. C.

Most elderly patients are on at least four medicati...

3. B.

The GEMS Diamond includes **G**eriatric patients, **E**nvironmer... assessment, **M**edical assessment, **S**ocial assessment.

4. A.

Dementia typically presents as a slow, progressive, irreversible deterioration in mentation.

5. D.

Alzheimer's disease is the most common cause of dementia.

CHAPTER 27

1. B.

Two-thirds of domestic violence patients have injuries to the face, neck, head, or arms.

2. C.

Cystic fibrosis is an inherited disorder that affects the lungs and digestive system.

3. A.

Most developmental disorders affect the CNS.

4. C.

DOPE stands for **D**isplacement, **O**bstruction, **P**neumothorax, **E**quipment malfunction.

5. A.

The first action for a patient with a ventilator malfunction should be to ensure adequate ventilation with a BVM.

Answers to Review Questions

CHAPTER 28

1. **B.**

   Emergency vehicle operators are permitted to disregard most traffic laws while responding to an emergency; however, you must always exercise due regard for safety.

2. **A., D.**

   Ambulance operators can disregard most traffic laws while in emergency mode; however, you should never pass a school bus with its stop sign extended, cross railroad tracks with the gates down, or speed through a school zone.

3. **A., D., E.**

   Safety during an emergency response is the priority, not speed. Practice defensive driving skills at all times.

4. **C.**

   The landing zone should be at least 100′ × 100′ at night and at least 75′ × 75′ during the day.

5. **B.**

   To reduce the risk of fatigue:

   - Limit shift work to 24 hours or less.
   - Use surveys to measure and monitor personnel fatigue.
   - Allow personnel to nap on duty.
   - Provide education in fatigue risk management.

CHAPTER 29

1. **B.**

   NIMS recommends either a unified command or a single command structure to avoid duplication of effort and freelancing.

429

Appendix

2. **A.**

    Clear text communication (no radio codes) is recommended on multiagency incidents.

3. **D.**

    The safety officer has the authority to stop any incident deemed an immediate life threat.

4. **A.**

    EMS tasks fall under the operations section.

5. **B.**

    Triage is intended to sort patients and determine the appropriate use of resources.

CHAPTER 30

1. **B.**

    Cribbing (usually wood pieces) is used to create a solid base of support to prevent collapse or shifting.

2. **A.**

    Phosgene and chlorine are pulmonary agents.

3. **D.**

    Leather gloves should be worn over PPE gloves when working around glass, sharp objects, or rope.

4. **B.**

    The minimum safe distance from an undeployed driver's side airbag is 10".

5. **C.**

    Blue: health hazard; Red: fire hazard; Yellow: instability; White: specific hazard; 4 (health hazard) = deadly.

Also Available from REA...

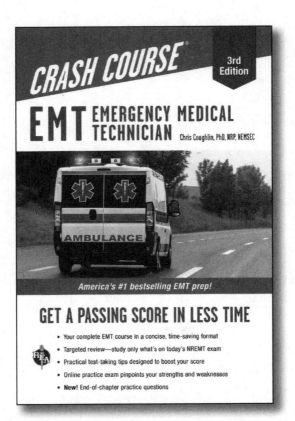

Research & Education Association
For more information, visit www.rea.com